FIRST TIME
MOM'S HEALTHY
EATING GUIDE
—— & ——
PREGNANCY
COOKBOOK

Prenatal Nutrition Journal, Meal Plans, Real Food & Delicious Recipe Must Haves for the New Expectant Pregnant Mother

MEGHAN PARKES

FIRST TIME MOM'S HEALTHY EATING GUIDE & PREGNANCY COOKBOOK

PRENATAL NUTRITION JOURNAL, MEAL PLANS, REAL
FOOD & DELICIOUS RECIPE MUST HAVES FOR THE
NEW EXPECTANT PREGNANT MOTHER

MEGHAN PARKES

COPYRIGHT

without the written contractual consent of the author and publisher.

TRADEMARK NOTICE

Any and all trademarks contained within this publication are the property of either the author and/or publisher and are not to be reproduced without specific written consent.

WANT FREE ACCESS TO THE COLORED VERSION OF THIS BOOK?

Scan the QR Code below to obtain the Free Colored versions in PDF and Epub (for reading on Kindle, iPad, iPhone, Android, Windows Phone, Nook, eReaders, Tablets, or PC)

CONTENTS

SPECIAL BONUS!

Want These 2 Bonus Books for FREE?

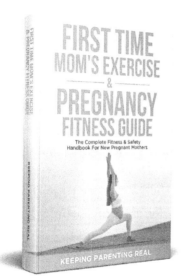 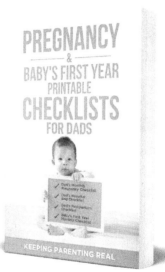

Get FREE, unlimited access to these and all of our new books by joining our community!

SCAN w/ your
QR code reader
TO JOIN!

Or Join @
KeepingParentingReal.com
/Pages/Free-Books

FEEDBACK

I would really appreciate your feedback and thoughts on the book. I welcome any positive comments or even any possible suggestions to improve the book for future editions. Please, don't be shy, let us know your thoughts at: Support@KeepingParentingReal.com

OTHER BOOKS IN THE SERIES

Keeping Parenting Real will be adding additional books to this pregnancy and parenting series over time, so keep an eye out!

The next instalment of the Pregnancy series covering your *'Baby's First Year'* will be out soon!

If you would like to join our private mailing list to be notified of new release books, simply email us at : Support@KeepingParentingReal.com

In the meantime, check out the latest releases from Keeping Parenting Real by Meghan Parkes and Aaron Edkins!

First Time Dads Weekly Pregnancy Guide
And
First Time Moms Pregnancy Guide
40 Things You Must Do, Before You're Due'

www.KeepingParentingReal.com/pages/library

Scan the QR Code

with your phone

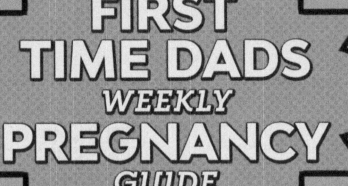

FIRST TIME DADS
WEEKLY
PREGNANCY
GUIDE

A Must-Have
Pregnancy Journal
for THE NEW DAD,
MOMS & PARENTS TO BE.

- ✓ Track Baby's Development & Mom's Changes
- ✓ Understand Your Feelings & How To Support Mom
- ✓ Monthly Checklists, Stories & Illustrations

Keeping Parenting
REAL

AARON EDKINS & MEGHAN PARKES

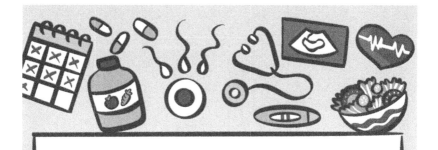

FIRST TIME MOMS
PREGNANCY GUIDE

Discover 40 Things You <u>MUST DO</u>
Before You're Due

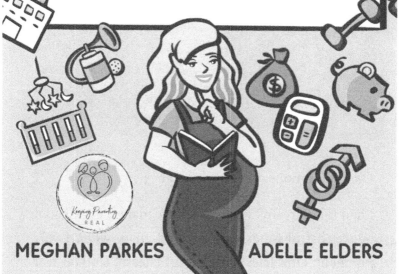

MEGHAN PARKES   **ADELLE ELDERS**

INTRODUCTION

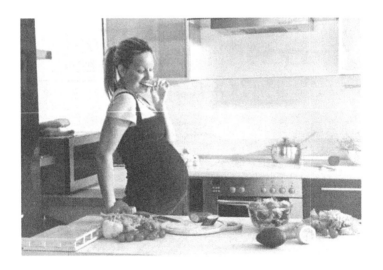

Congratulations on your pregnancy!

I had food dreams when I was pregnant. I even had a bucket list of foods that I would enjoy when I was pregnant: chili fries with lots of cheese! Do you feel me? I was ready to splurge and use all those "extra" calories that were now assigned to me because I was eating for two of course.

I felt so alive because now I could eat an unlimited amount of ice cream because isn't it made of milk? I need milk! Brilliant! Even though I was so nauseous, I ordered milkshake after milkshake. All the flavors you could dream of. The banana caramel milkshake at Sonic earned a special place in my heart.

Chugging my milkshake before my next pregnancy appointment, I started to feel a bit guilty. Then at my appointment, I stepped on the scale and I went into shock. I won't even tell you the shocking amount of weight that I gained.

My nurse-midwife gasped as she wrote the weight into my chart. And then we had the "talk". She didn't scold me but she went over the nutritional requirements that I needed to follow and then she firmly said that sugar was not a nutrient. Really?

Then came the concept of eating for two. The amount of "extra" calories was not as many as I had envisioned. In fact, I was way, way off. I left my appointment scared and frustrated. Another diet that I had to follow. I wasn't off the hook. I had to not only watch what I was eating but I had to eat foods that weren't usually in my diet to accommodate the nutrients that my baby needed to grow.

As that panic set in, I realized that there were many things I couldn't control about my pregnancy. I tried not to have a meltdown. Instead, I knew that in order not to feel so helpless, I could focus on what I do have control over - my pregnancy diet.

I put down those celebration milkshakes and rushed to the store to stock up on healthy food! But hold on! I didn't know what to shop for.

I know that to some women nutrition is a no-brainer for them? They put themselves on a high nutrient diet when they were trying to conceive. For others, good nutrition is a way of life. But that was different for me.

I didn't even know what foods to avoid during my pregnancy. I also didn't know what foods to include into my diet during my pregnancy. I knew I had to learn but where was I going to get this information?

Your pregnancy requires that you eat various nutrients that will sustain your pregnancy. Eating healthy is more than just going down a list of foods and making sure you eat what's on the list. You must know why you need those specific nutrients for your baby.

There's so much to learn about healthy eating during pregnancy, you may feel that you need to go back to school. At the very least, you may feel so over-whelmed you don't know where to turn.

Good news! Everything you need to know about your pregnancy diet is in this book.

Learn the following about your pregnancy and nutrition:

- What foods you should eat while you are pregnant.
- What nutrients you should include in your pregnancy diet.
- What foods you should avoid while you are pregnant.
- Plus, there is a bonus chapter of recipes, tips for healthy snacks, and also suggestions for pregnancy meal-planning!

My advice to you is to get a trough installed in your dining room . . .

Just joking! You don't need a trough. You need information because as you know: information is power! And boy does this book have information!

This book will never replace the advice and knowledge of your provider or a certified dietician. However, the more you know, the more you can discuss and query (your doctor and yes, ultimately Google).

So, get comfortable and read this book. It may just be the most important read of your pregnancy. Happy reading!

1

YOUR PREGNANCY DIET

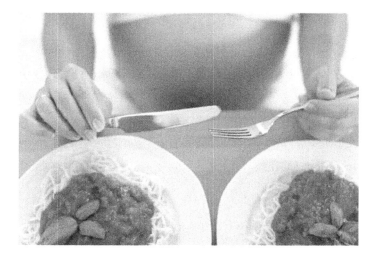

O nce upon a time, pregnant women were told that they were eating for two. This was like raising the checkered flag and starting an everything-goes buffet race. Pregnant women everywhere began to serve themselves twice. Foods that were once forbidden like ice cream, doughnuts, and other carbohydrates were feasted upon with the battle cry, "I'm eating for two!"

Then came the Age of Enlightenment, and obstetricians all over the world announced that although pregnant women always feel hungry, there is no need to eat for two. Pregnant women all over the world began to sob. The one bonus of pregnancy had been removed. From here on out, the guidelines were as follows:

If you are at a healthy weight when you get pregnant you don't need more calories in your first trimester. Good news, in your second trimester you need an extra 340 calories a day and 450 extra calories in the third trimester. (Miles, n.d.)

I know it's not a lot, but the most important thing is that you stay away from banana splits and Big Macs. The extra calories just give you a chance to consume more healthy nutrients.

If you are underweight or overweight when you start your pregnancy consult with your doctor about what your calorie goals should be.

I was obese during my last pregnancy and my doctor helped me to determine how many extra calories I should add to my diet. I am proud to say that I gained a healthy amount of weight and pretty much stayed at a stable weight for all of my pregnancy. If I can stay away from McDonald's or any of the other splendid fast-food joints near me, you can too!

WHAT TO STAY AWAY FROM

You must stay away from processed foods, sugary desserts, and packaged snacks. You might want to go through your pantry and your fridge and throw out these kinds of foods. Yes, your refrigerator needs a detox. Shall we send it to rehab?

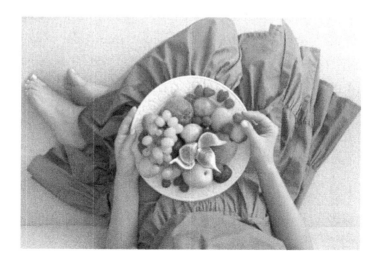

HEALTHY FOOD ALTERNATIVES

This doesn't mean you have to be stoic and avoid all the things that taste good in life. Step off the ledge and realize that there are many healthy food alternatives that you can incorporate into your pregnancy diet.

Fill your "sober" refrigerator with the ingredients for banana smoothies, all-fat nonfat sorbets, and plenty of fruits. Get to know things like agave syrup and other healthy sweeteners.

THE NAUGHTY FOOD RELAPSE

There will be days that you relapse. Someone, no names (your husband) will put something sweetly dangerous into your fridge like a triple fudge Blizzard or Sonic cookies and cream Blast. What are you to do? That's up to you but don't beat yourself up about it, just don't jump in your car every day at 3 pm for an ice cream treat. Let these little tastes of heaven be an exception and not the rule.

THE PREGNANCY FOUR-LETTER-WORD

And remember that the word "diet" does not always mean that you should go to an extreme and go on a weight loss diet. Remember, you are piling up the nutrients. If you go on a weight loss diet, you will not only decrease calories but also nutrients like iron, folic acid, and other essentials, (Miles, n.d.)

Your pregnancy diet doesn't have to be grim. Get creative and you will find joy in your diet.

HELP, PLEASE?

Wouldn't it be great to have a nutritionist on speed dial during your pregnancy? Maybe your health plan will pay for you to see a nutritionist? Make sure and find out what your benefits are in relation to your pregnancy. Also, check for free resources that are available in your community. You may qualify for the Special Supplemental Nutrition Program for Women, Infants, and Children (WIC) program that will offer you monthly classes on pregnancy and nutrition. The hospital where you are having your baby may also offer classes on nutrition.

DRINK YOUR WATER!

If your pantry is filled with diet caffeinated drinks or bottles of undiluted fruit juice, "just say no."

While you are pregnant, you will need to drink 10, 8-ounce glasses of water, (Rochman, n.d.) And, even more if you are exercising or outside in the heat. So, buy several cute water bottles and proceed to drink lots of water. It's good for you.

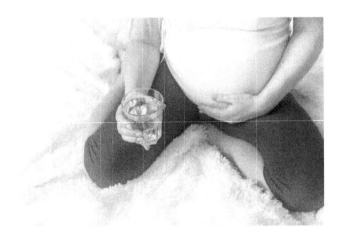

Water making you queasy?

If you just can't stomach water, I totally get you. I am a coke zero fanatic because of the bubbles and caffeine. What could be better when you are feeling so tired? The answer is not to depend on caffeinated sodas but to instead add flavor to your water like lemon or other citrus flavors. Also try infusing your water with fruit like oranges, apples, raspberries - any taste that you like. The taste will be subtle but refreshing.

Just remember that staying hydrated is very important.

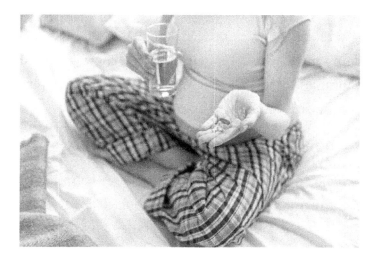

NEVER MISS YOUR PRENATAL VITAMINS

You promise that you will clean up your diet and fill your plate with the nutrients that you and your baby need. This is a good thing but what if you miss something? Some nutrients are very crucial and not having them in your diet could contribute to developing preeclampsia, neural tube defects (spina bifida), or low birth weight for your baby.

Let your prenatal vitamins do the heavy lifting! Take that vitamin every day as if your life depends on it. If taking that vitamin is unpleasant for you, talk to your doctor about other alternatives that you can take.

There are many choices in prenatal vitamins. Vitamins now come in mini form, chewable, and gummies. Find one that you like and take it every day like it's your new religion.

Mini-meals

As your pregnancy progresses and your baby grows, your digestive organs and your stomach are going to be crowded. Gone are the days when you could eat as much as you want. Now that your baby has invaded your body, you've got to trim those meals down so that you can be comfortable. Think mini-meals instead of full portioned meals.

Also eating mini-meals a little bit more often helps to keep something in your stomach at all times. This can help you maintain an even blood sugar level, (Rochman, n.d.).

Intelligent snack eating

Get rid of those processed snacks and start whipping up creative and cool snacks like out-of-this-world smoothies or overnight oatmeal. Think outside of the box and arm yourself with the best the world of natural food has to offer. Don't be armed and dangerous with highly processed food. Throw that beef jerky away and grab a bag of trail mix instead.

Remember that every bite you take, your baby takes too. Picture your baby in your womb with a jumbo beef jerky stick - what's wrong with that picture?

GET CREATIVE AND JUMP OUT OF THAT BOX

Let's be real here, the cravings are going to pull you to some really questionable foods. Let's talk about pizza and the fact that you have Pizza Hut and Papa John's on speed dial. Be honest with yourself and know that there will be pizza, burger, and fries cravings.

Don't despair, there is something you can do about this. Think outside the box and pile your pizza or burger with healthy ingredients. Try having an all-veggie pizza or a vegan burger. Instead of fries made from regular potatoes, try some oven-baked sweet potatoes instead.

2

ESSENTIAL PREGNANCY NUTRIENTS

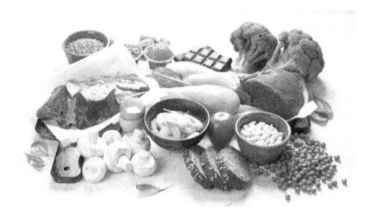

The minute you find out you're pregnant, your mind might wander and think about milk-shakes, ice cream, and any food on your forbidden list. Then two things happen: you begin to feel queasy, and your obstetrician gives you the "talk".

In my first pregnancy, the talk was about eating for two. At that moment, I didn't want to eat anything at all for the rest of my life, since I spent each morning sick like a dog and in the bathroom for longer than any person needs to be. But I was young, and I had hope. However, eating for two sounded great. I gained more than fifty pounds during pregnancy.

My second pregnancy was more of the same but by my third pregnancy, I had an obstetrician who was obsessed with pregnancy nutrition. When I gained weight after a remarkably successful Halloween, he gave me a serious talk. Sure, there were tears shed but it was the most important talk I ever needed to hear.

I learned that pregnancy nutrition is not about packing in the calories. Your daily pregnancy vitamin needs a little help, so it is important to pack in the right nutrients on your plate. In this chapter, we will explore the nutrients that every pregnant woman needs to consume.

Don't mind the calories too much. Instead, count nutrients because good nutrition is the best thing you can do for your baby. Your daily nutrition supports your pregnancy more than anything else you can do. Good nutrition can support the growth of your baby and even lower the risk of pregnancy complications like preeclampsia, anemia, and gestational diabetes. (Sinrich, 2020)

Being pregnant is a joyful time but it might be just a bit scary, to say the least. There is so much that you can't control about your pregnancy. It's natural to want to be the best for your baby. Eating well is a way to help your baby develop the best way possible. In a sense, you have control over something when you take charge of your nutrition.

You can't go wrong filling your plate with healthy foods. It's as easy as making good choices and avoiding bad choices. It's not rocket science. If I can do it, so can you.

Was I the poster girl of bad nutrition when I had my first two boys? I hate to admit it but "yes". I did get off of caffeine, but I ate whatever I was craving. And trust me I never craved salads or anything that was really healthy.

CRAVINGS: THE GOOD AND BAD NEWS

Oh yes, the cravings! How are you going to manage to be a healthy eater when that little person inside of you sends up an order for chili fries or something else more decadent like turtle cheesecake?

I'm happy to tell you that 50 to 90 percent of pregnant women have cravings, (Geddes, 2021). Think about that number: you are not alone! And it's not just craving a certain food or meal, some women have weird cravings that are beyond understanding. During the ninth month of my first pregnancy, I put catsup on my potato salad and used giant Fritos to scoop it up with. I figured at that point what did I have to lose? Hello! Baby is still developing! So mom, watch those cravings.

Reverse cravings

Cravings can also work a different way. Some moms experience an aversion to foods they particularly liked before pregnancy. I once prayed during my 3rd pregnancy for an aversion to ice cream and cheesecake.

A reverse craving can be really intense. I could not stand the smell of taco meat. My sense of smell was so sharp, I could smell the taco meat cooking when I was outside getting out of my car. I couldn't even look at a taco without dry heaving.

Reasons for pregnancy cravings

Mom's usually experience cravings at the end of their first trimester, with a peak that happens in the second trimester and a downturn during the third trimester, (Geddes, 2021) Don't worry if you are different Mom. Everybody has their own situation going on. You could be experiencing severe morning sickness into your second trimester, for example.

Here are some reasons for cravings:

- Pregnancy hormones
- Sensitive sense of smell/taste receptors
- Crossed nutrition signals
- A desire for comfort food

(Geddes, 2021)

These all make sense:

- Pregnancy hormones are awash in your body and they tend to change things up in your body.
- Your senses are on overdrive. Food that you love could taste horrible thanks to over-sensitive taste receptors or your super-sensitive nose.

- Your pregnant body may be craving things that it needs.
- Childhood comfort food like your mother's chicken and dumplings could be the one thing that makes you feel better.

Dangerous cravings

Cravings can be a scary thing if you crave something outside of your lifestyle. Like craving bar-be-que, if you are a vegan. Also, be aware that there is a medical condition called 'pica'. Pica happens when you crave non-foods like laundry starch, clay, dirt, and ashes. You can also have severe cravings for ice cubes. If this happens to you, call your doctor so that they can determine if there is a nutritional deficiency in your body. (Geddes, 2021).

I'm happy to tell you that in my 3rd, 4th, and 5th pregnancy, I had a better understanding of nutrition during pregnancy. The rest of this chapter will highlight the nutrients that are "must-haves" during your pregnancy. When you know what nutrients you need to include, you have a better idea of what you need to fill your plate up with. Let's get to it.

FOLIC ACID

Folic Acid (vitamin B9) is the rock star of pregnancy nutrients. Folic acid is important to the development of your baby. Folic acid is important in the first few weeks of pregnancy because some birth defects are developed during early pregnancy, (Sinrich, 2020). However, folic acid is good to have throughout your pregnancy as it lowers the chances of heart defects, preterm birth, and gestational diabetes.

Folic acid and pregnancy

The reason folic acid is so important during pregnancy is because it aids the body in creating protein and breaking it down. Folic acid helps in the formation of your baby's circulatory system and your baby's heart. Also, folic acid is instrumental in the role of creating DNA. In early pregnancy, folic acid plays a role in reducing the risk of spina bifida and other neural tube disorders. (Sinrich, 2020).

Your prenatal diet will include folic acid, or you can take a folic acid supplement. 400mcg per day is the recommended starting dose. It's wise to start this dose a month before you conceive. During pregnancy, it is recommended that you have between 400 to 600 mcg daily.

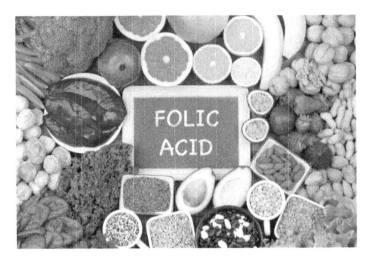

High food sources of Folic Acid

Oranges	Kidney beans
Fortified breakfast cereals	Green leafy vegetables
Beets	Strawberries
Cauliflower	

VITAMINS, MINERALS, AND PROTEIN

Vitamins and minerals are classed as micronutrients, which means you only need small amounts to satisfy your body's needs. Protein is a macronutrient, so you need this in much larger amounts. For a good nutritious diet, you should have a mix of these elements to help your baby develop and keep you in good shape during your pregnancy.

Vitamins

Vitamins are an important part of anyone's diet but during pregnancy they take on a more vital role. What follows is a list of the most important vitamins for you and where you can find them in your daily diet.

Vitamin A

You may have heard of Beta-carotene, a primary form of vitamin A. Beta-carotene is most often connected with carrots. My mother always advised me to eat my carrots so that I could see better. Is this an old wives tale or is there any science behind this saying?

What we know for sure, is that vitamin A is a powerful nutrient. Vitamin A is fat-soluble and contains antioxidants that include retinol, retinal and retinoic acids that are vital to the following systems: immune, visual, reproductive, and caller systems.

Vitamin A and pregnancy

Turns out that vitamin A is extremely critical to the development of your baby. It is the go-to vitamin for helping cell growth and division. Think of your baby's cells, bones, skin, and eyes and the rapid development that happens during your nine months of pregnancy. Vitamin A is critical to this development.

High Food sources of Vitamin A

Oranges	Kidney beans
Green leafy vegetables	Fortified breakfast cereals
Beets	Strawberries
Nuts	Cauliflower

Vitamin B6 (pyridoxine)

Vitamin B6 is a water-soluble vitamin that is especially important to the synthesis of neurotransmitters like serotonin and norepinephrine and myelin formation. Consequently, vitamin B6 is especially important to the brain.

B6 and pregnancy?

Just like vitamin B6 is essential to your brain, it is important to your baby's developing brain and nervous system. Vitamin B6 can also be a great help to your pregnancy. How? It's a definite first-trimester lifesaver when it comes to pregnancy nausea and vomiting, (Sinrich, 2020). When I found this out, I saw the hand of God.

High food sources of vitamin B6

Sunflower seeds	Pistachios
Tuna	Poultry
Prunes	Spinach
Lean beef	Avocado
Bananas	

Vitamin C (L-ascorbic acid)

You grew up knowing that vitamin C was important to you, but do you know why? Vitamin C is a water-soluble vitamin that aids in the production of collagen that is a vital protein. Why is collagen important? Collagen helps blood vessels, cartilage, tendons, and bones. Not only that but collagen bolsters immunity and helps with the absorption of iron. (Sinrich, 2021).

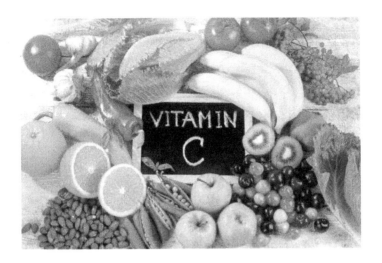

Vitamin C and pregnancy

Vitamin C helps your baby develop and some studies indicate low blood levels of vitamin C may bring about preeclampsia.

High food sources of vitamin C

Oranges	Broccoli
Strawberries	Green chilies
Red bell peppers	Guava
Papaya	Sweet Potatoes
Kale	Pineapple
Grapefruit	

Vitamin D

Was your mother a vitamin D fanatic? Was she always pouring you a glass of milk and insisting you drink it all? My mother read an article about vitamin D, and she discovered that it is produced in the skin when it is exposed to sunlight. Knowing this, she made sure I got enough play time outside.

Vitamin D is a fat-soluble vitamin that helps you to absorb calcium and maintain the normal mineralization of your bones. But the benefits of vitamin D don't stop there. It is also important to cell growth, the reduction of inflammation, and supporting a healthy immune system, (Sinrich, 2020).

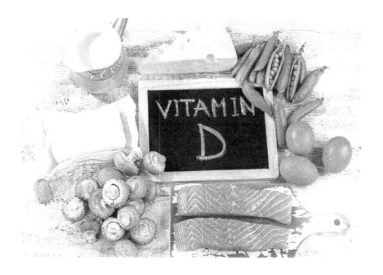

Vitamin D and pregnancy

Vitamin D is a big deal for your baby that is doing a lot of bone-building inside your womb. If you don't get enough vitamin D, your baby can develop rickets (softening of the bones) and muscle disease. There are even rare cases where babies have seizures when they are newborns, (Sinrich, 2020)

High food sources of vitamin D

Canned sardines in oil	Vitamin D-fortified milk
Carrots	Almonds
Eggs	

Riboflavin

Riboflavin or B12 as it is also known is an essential vitamin that helps the body make energy.

Riboflavin and pregnancy

Riboflavin does a lot for your baby's growth as it promotes healthy skin, bones, muscle, and nerve development, (Stewart, n.d.).

There is some evidence that a lack of riboflavin can put women at a greater risk for preeclampsia, (Stewart, n.d.)

High food sources of riboflavin

Milk	Eggs
Almonds	Chicken meat
Beef	Asparagus
Salmon	Cheddar cheese
Broccoli	

Thiamine (B1)

Thiamine or B1 is a water-soluble vitamin that is a part of the B vitamins

Thiamine and pregnancy

You and your baby need thiamine to convert carbohydrates into energy. This water-soluble vitamin helps the nervous system, muscles, and heart function. Your baby needs thiamine for brain development, (Steward, n.d.).

High food sources of Thiamine

Wheat germ	Peas
Brown rice	Pecans
Lentils	Oranges
Cantaloupe	Spinach
Eggs	Lean pork tenderloin
Whole wheat bread	Milk

Pantothenic acid (B5)

Pantothenic acid or B5 is a water-soluble B vitamin

Pantothenic acid and pregnancy

This vitamin is needed for the production of hormones and cholesterol. Pantothenic acid aids in the metabolism of carbohydrates, proteins, and fats. Pantothenic acids are essential to you and your baby as it is a component of coenzyme A (CoA) that is responsible for many chemical reactions in cells, (Stewart, n.d.)

High food sources of Pantothenic Acid

Beef liver	Sunflower seeds
Trout	Nonfat yogurt
Lobster	Avocado
Sweet potatoes	Milk
Chicken	Lean pork tenderloin
Egg	Feta cheese
Lentils	Split peas
Mushrooms (raw)	Whole wheat bread
Peanuts	Broccoli
Orange	

Phosphorus

Along with calcium, phosphorus is the most abundant mineral in our bodies. You can find 85% in your bones and teeth. No glowing in the dark, ok? Just stick to the phosphorus that is found in food.

Phosphorus and pregnancy

You and your baby need phosphorus for a lot of your bodily functions. Specifically, muscle movement, blood clotting, kidney, and nerve function along with tissue and cell repair, (Sinrich, 2020)

High food sources of Phosphorus

Salmon	Yogurt
Milk	Lentils
Almonds	Peanuts
Eggs	Whole wheat bread

Choline

Choline is a vitamin-like essential nutrient (Sinrich, 2020)

Choline and pregnancy

Involved in a lot of physiological processes like the production of neurotransmitters in the brain, choline is also needed for the production of phospholipids that helps the structure of cell membranes. Choline is good for aging brains, but you don't have to worry about that now (but just wait until you are raising teenagers!)

Some studies have found the intake of choline during your pregnancy can decrease the risk of neural-tube defects.

Choline is vital for fetal brain development and the memory center of the baby's brain.

High food sources of Choline

Salmon	Chicken
Broccoli	Cauliflower
Eggs	Lean beef

Minerals

Calcium

Calcium is a mineral in your body that is stored 99 percent in your bones and teeth. 1 percent of calcium is stored in your blood and soft tissues.

Calcium and pregnancy

Your baby needs calcium to develop your baby's bones and teeth. The most important thing for you to know about calcium and pregnancy is that your baby is getting calcium from your body. If you aren't getting enough calcium, your body won't let the baby go without and actually leeches it from your bones to give it to the baby. If this happens, it could lead to osteoporosis (brittle bones) in the future for you. (Sinrich, 2020).

There is an old wives tale that you lose a tooth for each baby that you have. This is remembered as the 'gain a child and lose a tooth' saying. So far there is no evidence that this is inherently the truth but maybe this tale has its basis in the bone leaching of calcium that happens when you don't have enough.

High food sources of calcium

Yogurt	Milk
Cheese	Calcium fortified orange juice
Salmon	Tofu
Sardines	Kale
Leafy Greens	Broccoli

Magnesium

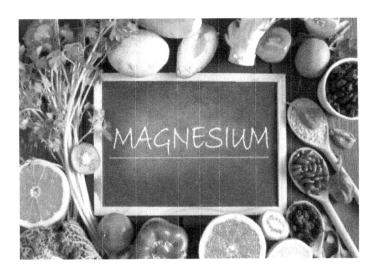

An essential mineral, magnesium regulates most of the systems in our bodies. One example of magnesium's importance to our bodies is that it relaxes and contracts muscles in conjunction with calcium.

Magnesium and pregnancy

Magnesium works to regulate insulin, control blood sugar levels, and stimulate enzyme function. If you don't get enough magnesium in your body, there is a chance that you will lack muscle strength and feel fatigued.

The benefits of magnesium for your baby are many but in particular, it strengthens your baby's teeth and bones. If you don't get enough magnesium, you risk poor fetal growth and preeclampsia.

High food sources for magnesium

Kidney Beans	Almonds
Peanuts	Peanut Butter
Black Beans	Edamame
Yogurt	Avocado
Spinach	

Zinc

Zinc is an essential trace mineral needed by your body in exceedingly small amounts. The main way zinc supports your body is to help the body's immune system fight invading bacteria and viruses. Also, your body needs zinc to help create proteins and DNA, (Sinrich, 2020)

Zinc and pregnancy

Zinc helps your baby's cell growth and developing genetic makeup.

During your pregnancy, it supports you in fighting off illnesses caused by invading bacteria and viruses. Can you believe that you don't get a break from catching a cold or a stomach virus when you are pregnant? If you manage your zinc intake, it can help to keep you from getting sick.

Consequences of not managing your zinc intake are low-birth-weight babies and problems during your labor and delivery.

High food sources for zinc

Baked beans	Almonds
Peanuts	Pork
Cashews	Lean beef
Yogurt	Dark turkey meat

Potassium

Potassium helps to maintain proper organ function. It is one out of seven macrominerals. (Sinrich, 2020)

Potassium and pregnancy

When you are pregnant, the fluid levels in your body increase a lot. Perhaps this is why I often had dreams of being a water balloon when I was pregnant? Potassium is an ingenious micromineral that works with sodium to help maintain a proper fluid balance in cells, (Sinrich, 2020)

Now that you don't feel like spending hours at the gym, potassium is your best friend as it helps maintain proper muscle tone. Plus, you might be able to say goodbye to aches, pains, and cramping thanks to maintaining the proper level of potassium in your body.

Moreover, potassium regulates your blood pressure. This is important because preeclampsia happens when your blood pressure is high.

High food sources of potassium

Bananas	Oranges
Prunes	Dried apricots
Peaches	Prunes
Carrots	Lentils
Wheat bran	Avocados
Pears	Lima beans
Sweet potatoes	Peas
Peanuts	

Copper

An essential trace mineral and micronutrient, copper helps your growth, and properly maintains the development and maintenance of your brain, organ and heart tissues, connective tissue, and bones.

Copper and pregnancy

Copper aids in creating your baby's heart, nervous immune, and skeletal systems and blood vessels, and cells.

During pregnancy your blood supply doubles, and your energy evaporates, copper can help you tolerate that doubled blood supply and diminishing energy level.

High food sources for copper:

Black pepper	Sunflower seeds
Hazelnuts	Cocoa
Whole grains	Prunes
Shiitake mushrooms	Lentils
Wheat bran	Cashews

Iron

A mineral that is part of the protein hemoglobin and lives in red blood cells is iron. An important function of iron is to transfer oxygen from the lungs to the tissues and return carbon dioxide from your tissues back to your lungs.

Iron also aids with the growth and development of cell function, and it builds hormones and connective tissues, (Sinrich, 2021)

Iron and pregnancy

Exhausted lately? Mom, you need more iron! Perhaps you need to date Ironman? Oh yes, I forgot, he's no longer in the Marvel Universe . . . Oh well.

To meet the increasing demands of iron for your body all you need to do is keep your iron consumption steady.

Why is iron in such demand? Both you and the baby need iron to help carry oxygen back and forth from mother to baby.

High food sources of iron

Edamame	Spinach
Chicken	Eggs
Kale	Beef
Beans	

Manganese

Is manganese a foreign language that you need to learn during your pregnancy when you travel to

Magnesia? Or is it a mineral that helps to convert macronutrients into usable energy? Correct answer: There is no need to learn the Manganese language or to travel to Magnesia.

Manganese and pregnancy

Day and night you are hard at work to create bone and cartilage for your baby and manganese helps you with that work. Manganese also helps with the metabolism of carbohydrates, cholesterol, and amino acids that help your baby grow to be the cutest baby ever. And if that isn't enough, manganese help protect the baby's brand-new cells from getting damaged, (Sinrich, 2020)

High food sources of manganese

Raisins	Bananas
Whole grains	Broccoli
Carrots	Oatmeal
Brown rice	Pecans
Legumes	Peanuts
Almonds	Pineapple
Spinach	Whole wheat bread

Chromium

A mineral that aids your body in breaking down fats, carbohydrates, and protein, chromium is definitely on the nutrient work crew that gets things done in your pregnant body.

Another important function of chromium is to help insulin maintain a normal level of glucose in your body. This function could be key to helping you if you develop gestational diabetes, (Stewart, n.d.).

Chromium and pregnancy

Your developing baby is working hard to grow tissues and chromium promotes this growth by helping the building of proteins in these tissues, (Steward, n.d.).

High food sources of Chromium

Broccoli	Bananas
Apples	Turkey Breast
Ham	Grapes
Potatoes	Bagels
Orange juice	

Iodine

Iodine is a trace element that is found in food, (Sinrich, 2021).

Iodine works hard with brain development and creating thyroid hormones. The normal function of the thyroid regulates the hormones that control core body function like metabolism, body temperature, and heart rate (Sinrich, 2021)

Iodine and Pregnancy

Your baby needs iodine for brain and nervous system development.

The World Health Organization (WHO) and the Centers for Disease Control and Prevention (CDC) have declared that the proper consumption of iodine can prevent the causes of intellectual disability in the world, (Sinrich, 2021).

High food sources Iodine

Milk	Plain yogurt
Tuna	Cod
Shrimp	Iodized table salt

Protein

Of all the nutrients in our body, protein may be the hardest worker. Protein is an amino acid that aids in building and repairing muscles when they are damaged. If that isn't enough protein builds bone, blood, nails, skin, and hair.

Feeling like you are on a rollercoaster of emotions? Maybe protein can help you out. Protein regulates hormones, enzymes, and chemical reactions in your body, (Sinrich, 2020).

Protein and pregnancy

Protein is very important in pregnancy because it is the building block of human cells. Think of that adorable baby and the cute little face and body that is growing inside of you. These cute features are brought to you by protein, the building block of human cells.

In the middle of your pregnancy, protein helps in the building of your baby's organs. So, make sure and keep that protein consumption steady. Also, you need to take B6 daily so that it can help break protein down in your pregnant body, (Sinrich, 2020).

High food sources of protein

Yogurt	Meat
Poultry	Eggs
Milk	Beans
Cheese	Nuts

These are the nutrients that are important for your pregnancy diet. To know if you are generally eating enough of the specific foods to meet the recommended requirements, keep a food journal with amounts so that your obstetrician or nutritionist can examine it.

MORE ESSENTIAL PREGNANCY NUTRIENTS

Avocado: the green hero fruit

Avocado is so much more than a guacamole dip. You can mash it up and add it to your sandwiches and say goodbye to mayo. It's a tough break up but don't worry avocado is sinfully delicious.

When you are hit with morning sickness, try some creamy avocado to soothe the beast. Avocados are full of folate and vitamin B6 that help your baby develop healthy tissue and brain growth, along with taming your morning sickness, (Taylor, 2020).

Embrace your new fruit hero; the avocado and do a happy dance as you mash it into culinary perfection.

The soybean pod of your dreams

Edamame is a cooked soybean pod that rivals the legume as a tasty source of protein. One cup has 18 grams of protein, 100 milligrams of calcium, 3.5 milligrams of iron, and 482 micrograms of folate. WOW!

Edamame is very easy to cook. If you buy them frozen, you can steam or microwave them, and they will be ready to eat in a few minutes. Add a little bit of salt or low sodium soy sauce and you've got a great snack.

You can also add them to a salad or puree them and add lemon juice and oil for a very creamy protein spread on your sandwiches.

Color your world

Very colorful vegetables are good choices for your pregnancy diet. Think green, red, orange, yellow, and purple fruits, and vegetables. Each color group brings with it a variety of vitamins and minerals, (Dougherty, 2020). So, get your color on and make your plate gleam with the technicolor wonder of fruits and vegetables.

Other nutrition superstars

- Nuts: they are chocked full of magnesium, zinc, potassium, vitamin E, protein, and fiber. They are also portable. Fill your pockets with nuts, it's the new have-to-have accessory.
- Almonds: packed with calcium
- Peanuts: packed with folate
- Walnuts: packed with omega-3 fatty acids
- Carrots: provide you with beta-carotene that is converted to a vitamin for your eyes. Oh, so good for your baby's developing eyes, skin, and organs.
- Red bell peppers: a big source of vitamin C and a healthy dose of fiber.

- Mangoes: a great source of vitamins like A and C. Mango salsa anyone?
- Eggs: 6 grams of protein in every egg, plus 44IU of vitamin D. Eggs: the new penny protein.
- Kale: the pregnancy superfood that contains folate, iron, vitamin C, calcium, vitamin A, E, and K, plus lots of fiber. Throw away those forbidden potato chips and toss some kale with olive oil and bake. Presto! Healthy chips.
- Oats: 25-30 grams of fiber and you are one regular pregnant lady. Further, oats can help your baby build healthy bones and teeth because it contains 30% of your daily magnesium needs.
- Bananas: rich in potassium that will help you keep a healthy blood pressure and manage your pregnancy bloat. Feeling tired and rundown? One banana can go a long way in boosting your energy level. Try one and conquer that pregnancy zombie that lives inside of you.
- Sweet Potato: 400% of vitamin A. What's not to love? Eat a sweet potato and get your baby's cells to divide at warp speed so that

they can become organs and other body parts.

- Quinoa: A whole grain that gives you 8 grams of protein, 5 grams of fiber, and close to 3 grams of iron per cooked cup. Also, sweet potatoes provide you with small amounts of calcium, magnesium, potassium, and zinc (Taylor, 2020)

- Low-fat milk: calcium, vitamin D, iodine, and protein are gifts that an 8-ounce glass of milk brings to you. The calcium in low-fat milk helps to bolster the development of the baby's bones and teeth. A single serving provides you a third of the calcium that you need per day.

- Dried fruit: it's like sweet candy on steroids. Dried fruit provides fiber, calcium, potassium, iron, and antioxidants.

- Whole grains: high in fiber, B vitamins, iron, folic acid (fortified) magnesium, Vitamin E, and selenium. And don't forget the phytonutrients, plant compounds that protect cells, (Dougherty, 2020)

- Greek yogurt: twice the protein of regular yogurt and an awesome source of probiotics, B vitamins, phosphorus, and calcium.

- Leafy greens (spinach, Swiss chard): a superfood loaded with nutrients like vitamin A, C, K, calcium, iron and folate, fiber, and antioxidants.
- Legumes (peas, peanuts, and beans): high in protein, iron, folate, potassium, and magnesium.

And while you are eating all these delicious nutrient-rich foods, don't forget to drink your water. It's important to keep hydrated because dehydration can increase the risk of early labor, (Taylor, 2020)

FOLLOWING A VEGETARIAN DIET WHEN YOU ARE PREGNANT

Many might ask if it is safe to follow a plant-based protein diet when you are pregnant. The answer is: yes, of course.

If being vegetarian or vegan is already a lifestyle choice for you, chances are you are already a pro at getting all your vital nutrients. If you want to follow a plant-based diet for the first time, learn how you can get all your pregnancy nutrients from other sources other than animals.

Also, let your obstetrician or midwife know that you are following a diet of alternate proteins so that they can determine if you need added vitamins or supplements.

The bonus of a plant-based diet

There are some great benefits to following a plant-based diet. Here are a few of them:

- An abundance and variety of vitamins, protein, and minerals built into your diet
- Lots of fiber
- Low in saturated fat and cholesterol

Upgrade your food plan

Some plant-based diets offer a little flexibility. You might feel that you need this when you are pregnant. Here are some examples of these diets:

- Lacto-Ovo vegetarian diet - includes egg and diary
- Lacto vegetarian diet - includes dairy
- Ovo vegetarian diet - includes eggs
- Pescatarian diet - includes seafood
- Flexitarian diet – you choose to be flexible

and include some animal protein into your diet once in a while.

Let's be truthful, your pregnancy diet is really an undercover flexitarian diet as you try to manage your cravings and include all the foods that you need into your meal plan.

Overall, if you want to follow a vegan/vegetarian diet, you don't need to worry that it is not good for your baby. Just incorporate the extra minerals, vitamins, and protein into your diet, and with some careful monitoring from your healthcare provider, you can make this special diet work.

3

AVOIDING NUTRITIONAL DISASTERS

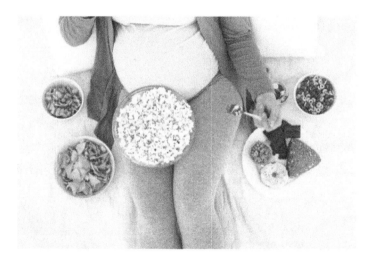

Danger seems to lurk everywhere when you are pregnant. What are you to do? Lock yourself up in a safe room until your due date? If you do opt for this solution, make sure you don't take any sushi, raw meat, deli meat, and unpasteurized cheese with you! Why?

All of these foods carry the risk of having bacteria that can make you sick. So put down that turkey slice and run screaming from the deli! Calm down, I am just kidding around. You don't have to run but step lively and get out of that deli - now!

I know you won't be eating raw meat, unless you have some kind of weird craving and unpasteurized cheese is easy to avoid. Just read the label of your cheese and make sure it is pasteurized - easy fix.

Food poisoning

You never think that you will have a health violation in your kitchen, but it can happen. You may not get a health rating from an inspector, but food safety needs to be a priority in your kitchen, especially when you are carrying precious cargo.

Let's review how to store food safely:

Storing your food

Is it necessary to keep the temperature in your refrigerator at arctic zone levels? No, you really don't have to keep it so cold that a snowstorm in your fridge can happen at any time. The suggested temperature for your refrigerator is 35 to 40 degrees Fahrenheit. Your freezer can be set at below zero, (Miles, 2021). Keeping your refrigerator set at the correct temperature can help your food not become contaminated by disease-causing organisms.

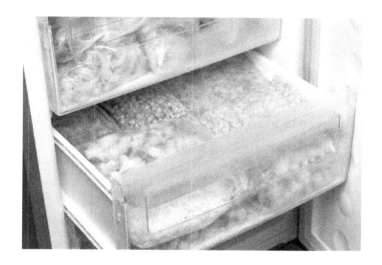

Ben Franklin had a saying,

"Guests, like fish, begin to smell after three days."

— BEN FRANKLIN

The food in your fridge are guests in your home, keep track of its arrival date so that you can figure out when that food needs to depart into the trash can. You might feel guilty throwing out food that seems perfectly fine but STOP! You are pregnant and you really need to pay attention to proper food storage to stave off the chance of getting food poisoning.

Prepare with care

Once you've aced the storage issue, it's time to make sure that your food is prepared with care. Do the following:

- Avoid contaminating food by using separate cutting boards, utensils, and plates for eggs, seafood, and raw meats (Miles, 2021).
- Wash all your produce and peel all your vegetables and fruits before eating them. And contrary to your instincts, don't rinse eggs, poultry, or meats as this can further spread bacteria.
- Cook all your food thoroughly. Get into the habit of using a food thermometer to test for doneness. For example, meat needs to be cooked at 165 degrees Fahrenheit and whole

poultry should be 18 degrees Fahrenheit in the thigh to ensure that it's cooked thoroughly. And don't go sampling your food until it is fully cooked.

- When you reheat make sure that you heat all leftovers to 165 degrees Fahrenheit. The listeria bacteria is a cold stone survivor and can continue to grow in your refrigerator. By reheating to 164 degrees F or until the food is steaming hot, you can kill the listeria that lurks within.

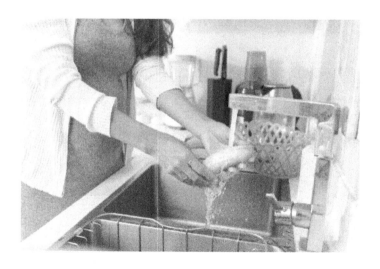

Cleanliness is next to Godliness

If you are not a cleaning fanatic coming into your pregnancy, now is the time to catch that cleaning bug. Always wash your hands with hot soapy water for at least 20 seconds. Wash utensils and surfaces with hot soapy water. Consider everything to have been in the contamination zone and treat accordingly.

And even though it's a pain, clean that refrigerator! Remember that listeria can survive in a cold fridge and can continue to grow (at a slow rate). Catch that bug (the cleaning bug) and scrub everything down with hot soapy water. You don't need an industrial-strength cleaner as a mild liquid dishwashing detergent like Dawn will suffice, (Miles, 2021)

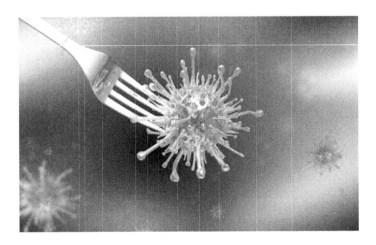

Lastly, wash those dishcloths and dish towels on a regular basis in very hot water, (Miles, 2021). Evict all the dangerous bacteria simply by washing dish towels in your washing machine. If you use sponges to clean your kitchen, don't get too attached. Even if you microwave the sponges, you aren't going to kill all the bacteria that love to reside on the sponge. Just throw those sponges away frequently for the love of God. No long-term attachments, please.

Overall, kill the bacteria in your kitchen using all methods available. You and your baby need to remain safe from food poisoning.

4

WHAT'S SAFE AND WHAT'S NOT

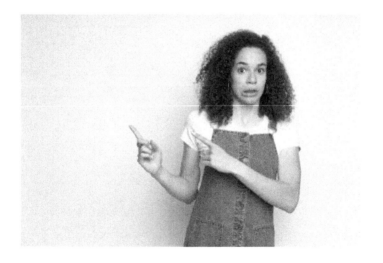

I n the previous chapter, I told you not to eat raw
meat. But what about the sushi or the deli meat?
What's wrong with those two foods?

Listeria is what is wrong with these foods. What is listeria? It sounds like some off-brand mouthwash, doesn't it? In truth, listeria is a bacteria fully named listeria monocytogenes. Although your chances of being infected with listeriosis are very low, your chances are higher during pregnancy, (Wu, 2020). And oh boy, can listeria cause problems.

If you eat contaminated food, your reaction could be severe or mild. Basically, you will feel like you have caught the flu. The symptoms are:

Muscle pain	Back ache
Headache	Fever over 100.6 (degrees F)
Gastrointestinal Symptoms like diarrhea	

(Wu, 2020)

You may have one or more of these symptoms or none at all. Contact your obstetrician if you suspect you have tangled with this troublesome bacteria. Even if your symptoms are mild, it's just always good to give your obstetrician a call.

If your obstetrician suspects you have a listeriosis infection, he will order a test and blood work to check if you have this bacteria in your system. Your obstetrician may also monitor your baby's health. If you are infected, your obstetrician may prescribe an antibiotic.

Don't worry so much about getting a listeriosis infection, the Centers for Disease Control and Prevention (CDC) estimates that in the United States, 1,600 people contract listeriosis every year. Only a sixth of the cases that get reported occur in women that are pregnant, (Miles, 2021)

Foods to avoid

Now that we have filled your head with the top foods to eat when you are pregnant, it is time that we give you a list of what to avoid when you are pregnant. Some of these foods and drinks, you know instinctively as a mother, that you should avoid. Some foods are not that obvious. Let's examine the foods that you should avoid.

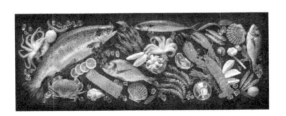

High-Mercury Seafood

The FDA and the EPA advise pregnant women to stay away from these fish due to the high levels of mercury that can impair your baby from developing a healthy brain and nervous system.

Limit canned solid white or albacore tuna to 6 oz. per week. (Roth, 2020)

This can be confusing, but you CAN have seafood that is low in levels of mercury and high in fatty acids like DHA, EPA (both forms of omega 3).

Some of the fish you can eat are:

Chilean sea bass	Grouper
Bluefish	Catfish
Salmon	Tilapia
Pantagonian toothfish	Mahi Mahi
Halibut	Carp

Other seafood you can eat:

Clams	Clams
Crabs	Crabs
Crawfish	Crawfish
Lobster (American and spiny)	Shrimp
(Miles, 2020)	

Can you eat meat during your pregnancy?

Meat is a high source of protein, so it is hard to avoid. The danger lies in eating meat that is under-cooked because it may contain the bacteria salmonella or the parasite toxoplasma. If you are exposed to this bacteria and parasite, you could be in for some serious health problems. Also, both of these bacteria and parasites can infect your baby. Yikes!

However, you can prevent this danger by cooking your beef, veal, pork, and lamb at 145 degrees Fahrenheit. If you are cooking ground meats, make sure they reach 160 degrees Fahrenheit and that poultry reaches 165 degrees F.

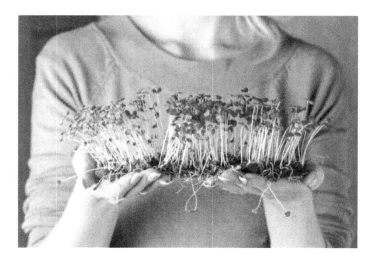

Hippie soul food: sprouts

Do you have the soul of a hippie or a health food nut? Time travel back to the 1970s to get one of those gorgeous vegetable protein sandwiches piled high with sprouts. Seems like those sandwiches would be perfect for a pregnant woman, right? Nope. Wrong!

Raw sprouts are not good for you because even before they are grown, if the seeds have a cracked shell, bacteria can grow there. And guess what, you generally eat sprouts raw so there is no way to kill that bacteria!

What to avoid

- Raw alfalfa
- Clover
- Radish
- Mung bean sprouts

So put away your bell-bottoms and stay away from raw sprouts.

Cheese is a great source of many things like calcium. In the US most soft cheese is made with pasteurized milk so you are good to go, (Roth, 2020.) But buyer beware, always check that soft cheese and make sure it was pasteurized.

Fancy cheese

Hope you aren't a cheese snob who loves artisanal or imported cheese. Why? It's the pasteurization issue again.

Stay away from these artisanal or imported cheeses:

Feta	Brie
Camembert	Fresh mozzarella
Blue Cheese	Limburger
Queso Blanco	Queso Fresco
(Roth, 2020)	

Liver

There's nothing like liver smothered with onions. Why don't they have it on some popular restaurant menus anymore? I know I won't dare cook it at home because let's be honest, it's a bit intimidating, all dark red and jelly-like. Okay, I'll stop with the horrific visualization.

Is liver good for you? Yes, it is but you've got to avoid it in your first trimester and limit it during pregnancy. Liver is nutrient-dense with vitamins, minerals, and proteins, (Bellenfonds, 2021). Yet the liver eventually overdoes it when it comes to vitamin A. In fact, liver contains a high concentration of this vitamin and that can be dangerous during pregnancy.

So, liver haters, you are off the hook. Liver lovers, slow down and count the livers. Don't overdo it. You can have half a serving (1.5 oz.) once or twice a month and for goodness sake, make sure it's cooked all the way, (Bellenfonds, 2021).

Eggs

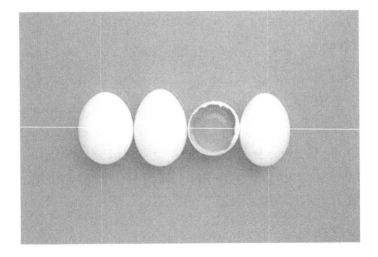

Eggs are safe to eat during your pregnancy as long as they are pasteurized and fully cooked. Don't go gathering fresh eggs in a basket and eating them, ok? Be safe.

The other condition for making eggs safe is that you don't eat any raw eggs. You are not Rocky Balboa, do not make yourself a power drink with raw eggs. Avoid the following types of egg dishes:

Poached eggs	Soft-boiled eggs
Eggs over medium	Eggs over easy

I don't mean to take your joy away but keep away from the following foods made with raw eggs:

Homemade dressings	Caesar salad dressing
Hollandaise Sauce	Homemade Ice Cream
Mouse	Meringue
Tiramisu	Raw batter
Cookie dough	Homemade eggnog

Keep those eggs fully cooked and pasteurized and you are good to go.

Chocolate during pregnancy

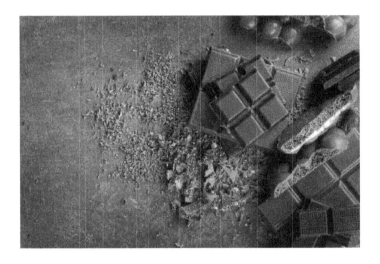

Let's get to what is really important: chocolate

Will you have to throw out your secret chocolate stash now that you are pregnant? Put away the trash can and the padlock, here are some facts about chocolate during pregnancy.

Chocolate is safe in moderation as there is evidence that chocolate could lower your risk of preeclampsia and gestational hypertension. There is also evidence that a daily dose of dark chocolate could improve blood flow to the fetus during the first trimester. How much chocolate can you eat? Around 54 chocolate chips or a quarter of a bar of chocolate.

Of course, there is always a Debbie Downer who says:

- Chocolate could contribute to unhealthy weight gains.
- Chocolate contains caffeine

Official guidelines

Here are some guidelines from the U.S. Department of Agriculture, the Department of Health and Human Services, and the American College of Obstetricians and Gynecologists.

- Limit added sugars and saturated fat to less than 10% of calories per day.
- Limit caffeine intake to below 200 milligrams a day.

(Miles, 2021).

Sadly, there are some conditions where it's highly suggested that you skip chocolate during pregnancy (gasp!)

- Your body can't control your blood sugar, (Prediabetes or diabetes).

- You have gestational diabetes.
- You're gaining too much weight.

(Miles, 2021)

Overall, girls, remember moderation when eating chocolate!

Peanut butter during pregnancy

Is Peanut butter a go or no-go during pregnancy? Good news - have as much peanut butter as you want! Yea! In fact, some studies say if you eat peanut butter during your pregnancy, your baby has a better chance of not developing a food allergy to peanut butter, (Boyd-Barret, 2021).

Peanut butter is a nutritious source of polyunsaturated fatty acids and antioxidants. Plus peanut butter has a lot of folates that decrease the risk of neural tube defects, (Boyd-Barret 2021).

Pour yourself a big glass of milk and enjoy that peanut butter and fruit spread sandwich! If peanut butter is not your fave, try other types of nut butter like almond or cashew.

Honey during your pregnancy

Honey is safe for you to eat while you are pregnant. If something goes south when you eat honey, your body can handle the bacteria in honey. Studies have shown that the bacteria from honey can not pass through the placenta and to your baby, (Boyd-Barret, 2021). Also, raw or unpasteurized honey is okay because it doesn't contain the risk of listeriosis like unpasteurized cheese or deli meats.

However, if you have the following it isn't a good thing to eat honey:

- Crohn's disease
- Gastrointestinal problems or abnormalities
- Inflammatory bowel disease
- Previous gastric surgery

(Boyd-Barrett, 2021)

A small caution: remember that honey is an added sugar so your intake ought to be no more than 6 teaspoons a day. If you have gestational diabetes, try to avoid honey.

Spicy food, MSG, and Artificial Sweeteners

Did you know that at 15 weeks, a baby's taste buds are fully formed? Baby is also swallowing amniotic fluids so it is very likely that they are tasting what you are eating, (Bellefonds, 2021). What you eat shapes your baby's food likes-dislikes.

Spicy food

You might question what spicy food tastes like for your baby or even if you should eat spicy food at all. It's a fact that spice boosts your overall health because the capsaicin (spicy chemical) in your peppers carry anti-inflammatory properties and can boost your immune system and heart health, (Bellefonds, 2021)

Here are some spicey facts:

- Expands baby's future tastes.
- A popular pregnancy food craving
- Doesn't help to trigger labor

MSG and pregnancy

Don't worry about the food additive, MSG, during your pregnancy. If you didn't have trouble with it before, you should be good to eat it when expecting as it doesn't put your baby at risk, (Hawthorn, 2021). So go ahead and order that Chinese take-out, I know you have it on speed dial.

Artificial sweeteners

The following sweeteners are approved as safe to have during pregnancy in moderation by the Food and Drug Administration:

Aspartame (NutraSweet and Equal)	Sucralose (Splenda)
Acesulfame Potassium	Neotame
Advantame	

Stevia is considered safe but it is not recognized to be safe by the FDA. Saccharin is also not approved by the FDA because studies have shown two things: it passes the placenta and can stay in baby's tissue and large amounts of saccharin may cause bladder cancer in rats. Human studies do not show this link, (Hawthorne, 2021).

Also, if you have a rare genetic disease called PKU (phenylketonuria) avoid aspartame.

If you do eat or drink something with saccharine, don't panic, it's okay. Just be careful not to ingest a lot of it.

Takeout, and buffet foods

The main concern when you eat buffets is that they are not prepared safely or kept at the proper temperature when they are in the buffet line. Unless you know for sure, don't eat at buffets.

Takeout food is safe as long as you know that the restaurant has a good health rating. Again, the concern is the preparation and storage of the food. Dangerous bacteria can develop if proper safety measures are not taken. So it's okay but be careful.

To drink or not to drink

Now that we've covered the best foods to eat when you are pregnant and what not to eat, what's left? Drinks, yes I am going to pick on what you drink now. It's obvious that you can't go on any late-night benders but what about caffeine, soda, water, and unpasteurized juice? Is it alright to guzzle juice? And what about water? Do you drink until you feel you are going to float out to sea?

Caffeine

My secret love when I was pregnant was sugar-free sodas with caffeine. The hardest thing to do was to quit my soda habit and limit my caffeine intake. Researchers at the National Institutes of Health and other research facilities have been trying to crack the pregnancy caffeine code. So far they have determined that women who drink less than 200mg of caffeine a day (half a cup of coffee) have slightly smaller babies than non - caffeine drinkers, (Lake, 2021)

Calm down, you can still have that cup or half a cup of coffee or can of soda - depending on the amount of caffeine they contain. Yes, there is math and reading in play here: read the labels to play the caffeine game. It's important to read labels or to investigate how much caffeine your coffee or soda may have.

There is no link in moderate caffeine consumption in pregnancy (less than 200 mg a day) to:

- Low birth weight
- IUGR
- Miscarriage
- Premature birth

(Lake, 2021)

So the motto with caffeine is moderation. Ask your obstetrician or midwife for any caffeine moderation tips they may have.

Unpasteurized drinks

First of all, you have two things to watch out for: unpasteurized drinks like fruit juice or on rare occasions milk or milk beverages that stay natural and unpasteurized and SUGAR.

Second, there are limits to everything you drink. Put down that red bull! I see you sliding that diet coke energy drink out of view. Drive on by that Starbucks!

Fun fact: Starbucks will fix you up a nice cold drink of water in their special sippy cups that save the world from plastic straws. If you have the willpower, stop by to order cold water. I know you can do it.

Third, soda is not your friend. Break up with it as soon as you find out you are pregnant. The real culprit is the sugar-loaded sodas that we enjoyed during our carefree youth.

Technically, sugar sodas can be had when you are pregnant but why drink all those empty calories?

And, why take a chance that your pregnant body will be able to process all of that sugar? Put down that Big Gulp and go for a much smaller drink size. Anybody for a mini-soda? They sell smaller cans of soda and there is such a thing as small. Hang in there and make good choices.

Pregnancy and water: cry me a river and just float away?

Water is very good for you when you are pregnant. Drink as much as possible. Your goal needs to be to stay hydrated each and every day. I get queasy if I have to drink plain water (unless it is ice cold from Starbucks, of course). Here are some drinks that can go towards your hydration quota:

Milk	Fruit and vegetable juices
Decaffeinated herbal teas	Raspberry tea
Sparkling or flavored waters	

Also, be aware that 20% of water intake comes from food sources, (Bellefond, 2020). Fruits that contain lots of water:

Watermelon	Cantaloupe
Pears	Strawberries

Tap water and bottled water safety

Do you know how safe your public water system is? Is it safe to drink tap water? For these answers, you might head to the internet or call your water board directly. Furthermore, bottled water should also be held to the same standards. Do an internet search on different brands of water and find out if contaminants have been found in that particular brand of bottled water.

Also note that water sold in bottles that contain BPA, a chemical that mimics estrogen, is not pregnancy-friendly, (Bellefond, 2020).

Alcohol and your pregnancy

The stress of being pregnant can make you feel like an afternoon or before bed cocktail would be nice. Back in the day, a little glass of wine or a martini with dinner was acceptable for a pregnant woman. I can see my hip pregnant mom with a cigarette and a martini in her hand. After all, it was 1965 and they still had twilight sleep when you went into labor.

Now things are different. Studies have been done and we have more information on the effects of alcohol on a fetus. Sad news, if alcohol is your party-go-to, it has been found that there is no safe amount of alcohol while you are pregnant, (Lake, 2021).

Even a small amount of alcohol could have detrimental effects on your baby. Think fetal alcohol syndrome, birth defects, and developmental problems. All these effects can be prevented by abstaining from alcohol, (Lake, 2021).

The CDC reports that 10% of pregnant women in the US say that they have had a drink while pregnant occasionally while 1/3 of the women report binge drinking.

The American College of Obstetricians and Gynecologists and the American Academy of Pediatrics say that pregnant women need to avoid alcohol completely, (Lake, 2021).

Don't be afraid to reach out for help if abstaining from alcohol is difficult. While pregnant, even though I wasn't a habitual alcohol imbiber, I went to a few AA meetings and the members there were so supportive and passed on great information that was very helpful. Also, your obstetrician will be able to get you in touch with help. Whether it is a helpful website or a counselor, don't be afraid to reach out.

So that's the skinny on what you should drink when you are pregnant. Go forth and stay hydrated!

THE JOY OF COOKING WHILE PREGNANT

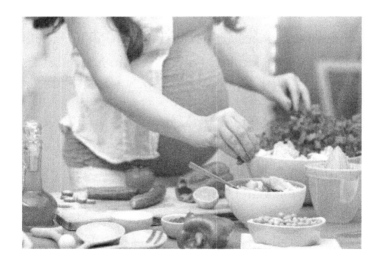

M aking sure that you fit all the recommended nutrients into your pregnancy diet can be very intimidating. How do you round up all these nutrients and fit them into a meal plan? How do you know when you have eaten enough of the recommended nutrients?

Sure, you could rise in the morning and start eating at a trough of fruits and vegetables but isn't there any easier way? Put up your feet and let's explore a couple of meal plans and a very special tool that can help you keep out of the trough.

HARVARD HEALTHY EATING PLATE

What you put on your plate during pregnancy starts with a meal plan. Harvard School of Public Health has created the Healthy Eating Plate to help mothers benefit from the latest research on balanced diets.

Harvard has a different take on what foods moms should eat when pregnant. Whole-grain foods, healthy vegetable oils, and a limit on milk and dairy products are out front and center for these meal plans. Avoiding processed meats totally, limiting red meat and refined grains like white bread and white rice are also important to the Harvard Healthy Eating Plate, (Montgomery, 2021).

If you were planning to have a big glass of Kool-Aid or soda pop, make other plans. The Harvard Eating Plate promotes drinking healthy amounts of water and skipping drinks loaded with sugar. Don't despair, infuse your water with fruit and there's a party in your glass. I know, it's not the same as a glass of Kool-Aid or fizzy soda but that's Harvard for you. Maybe your baby can include your suffering in his Harvard college admission essay?

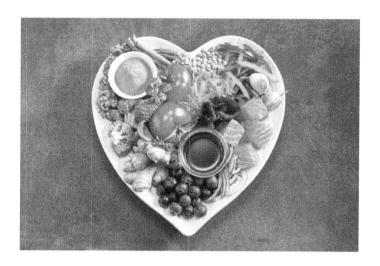

MY PLATE MEAL PLANS

Tired of building food and nutrition pyramids? Good news, the U.S. Department of Agriculture (USDA) has revised that food pyramid into a My plate system for you. They take all those categories off the pyramid and arrange them onto a healthy plate for you.

To make things easier on pregnant moms, there is even a special section where a pregnant or breast-feeding mom can personalize a tracking system that you can develop from your personal data. Age, height, pre-pregnancy weight, activity level, and what trimester you are in, are the data that this tracking system needs for developing your healthy plate, (Montgomery, 2021)

Once you get that system together, you can design your individualized meal plan. There will be guidelines for what food you should put on your healthy plate. If you are interested in this system, go to: ChooseMyPlate.gov.

SAMPLE FOOD PLAN

So, what do the Harvard and My Plate menus look like? Let's look at the My Plate healthy food requirements for pregnant moms. This plan was developed for a 32-year-old woman who is 5'4" and 130lbs pre-pregnancy weight. She is in her second trimester and gets 30 minutes of daily physical activity. This is the sample plan available on the USDA website. When you plug in your personal data, your plan will be different. Let's take a look at this suggested

Healthy Plate. The amounts are what you should have daily.

7 oz. Grains
2 cups of fruit daily
3 cups vegetables
6 oz lean protein and beans
12 oz. of fish

3 cups dairy
6 tsp. healthy fats and oils
266 discretionary calories
(Montgomery, 2021)

Remember that as you progress into another trimester, the food amounts will change.

Which meal plan is best?

These meal plans might not be easy for you but it's important to at least strive for these Healthy Plates. Either the USDA plan or the Harvard plan can be good for you. The most important thing is that you have some help in trying to get all your nutrients into your diet.

If you have the time and energy, you can develop your own healthy plate but if this isn't possible, these two programs are awesome tools for you to use.

A neonatologist and medical director of the March of Dimes notes that if you eat nutritiously when you are pregnant, you will have huge dividends for the rest of your baby's life, (Montgomery, 2021).

Exceptions to the rule

An important thing to note is that the Harvard and USDA healthy plates might not be for everyone. If you fit into one of these groups, it's important to follow your obstetrician's recommendations for your pregnancy meal plans.

Exceptions

- If you are overweight, you will need guidance on how to cut down your calorie intake.
- If you are underweight you will need guidance on how to increase your calorie intake.
- If you are a teenager, your nutrition requirements will be different.
- If you are expecting twins, triplets, or more!

your requirements will be very different from a mom expecting a single.

- If you develop gestational diabetes or if you are diabetic before pregnancy consult with a dietician for the best possible meal plan.

(Montgomery, 2021)

Overall, developing meal plans during pregnancy really helps you to get all those great nutrients into your diet. The idea of meal plans reminds me of the dinosaur years where you wrote down everything you ate on a scrap of notebook paper and prayed for the best.

MAKING PREGNANCY NUTRITION FUN

Go old school and refer to recipes to vary your nutrition plans. Believe me, it can get really old following the same sample menu over and over. This section will give you an amazing start to adding fun and nutritious food to your meal plan.

Let the fun begin!

A short message from the Author:

Hey, are you enjoying our pregnancy guide?
We'd love to hear your thoughts! ☺
Many readers do not realize how hard reviews are to
come by and how much they really help an author.
We would be incredibly grateful if you could take
just 60 seconds to write a brief review on Amazon,
even if it's just a few short lines!

Customer Reviews

⭐⭐⭐⭐⭐ 2
5.0 out of 5 stars ▾

5 star		100%
4 star		0%
3 star		0%
2 star		0%
1 star		0%

See all verified purchase reviews ›

Share your thoughts with other customers

Write a customer review

Simply visit:
www.Amazon.com/RYP

Your review will genuinely make a difference
and will help us gain exposure for our work.
Thank you in advance for taking the time to share
your thoughts!
☺

SPECIAL BONUS!

Want These 2 Bonus Books for FREE?

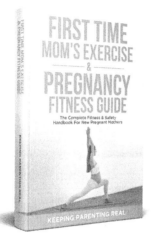 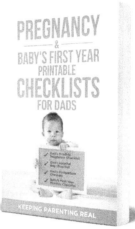

Get FREE, unlimited access to these and all of our new books by joining our community!

SCAN w/ your
QR code reader
TO JOIN!

Or Join @
**KeepingParentingReal.com
/Pages/Free-Books**

FEEDBACK

I would really appreciate your feedback and thoughts on the book. I welcome any positive comments or even any possible suggestions to improve the book for future editions. Please, don't be shy, let us know your thoughts at: Support@KeepingParentingReal.com

OTHER BOOKS IN THE SERIES

Keeping Parenting Real will be adding additional books to this pregnancy and parenting series over time, so keep an eye out!

The next instalment of the Pregnancy series covering your 'Baby's First Year' will be out soon!

If you would like to join our private mailing list to be notified of new release books, simply email us at : Support@KeepingParentingReal.com

In the meantime, check out the latest releases from Keeping Parenting Real by Meghan Parkes and Aaron Edkins!

First Time Dads Weekly Pregnancy Guide

And

First Time Moms Pregnancy Guide

40 Things You Must Do, Before You're Due'

www.KeepingParentingReal.com/pages/library

Scan the QR Code

with your phone

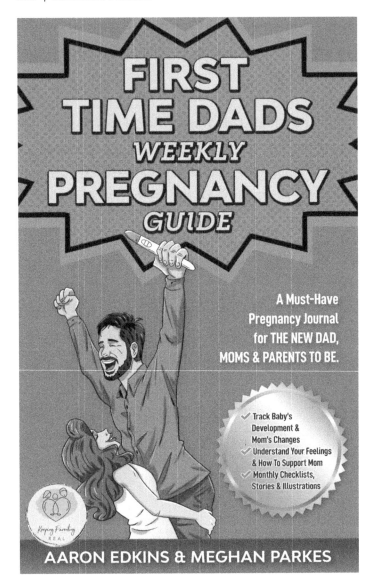

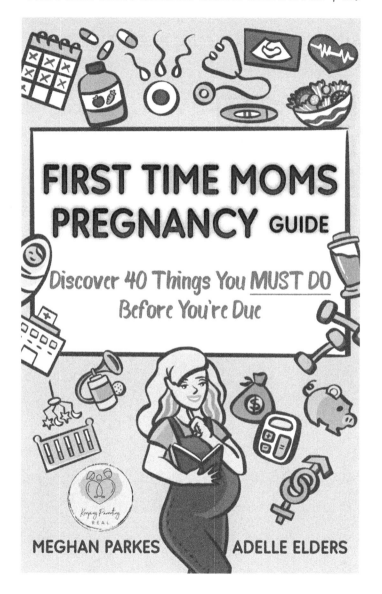

SUPPORT THE KEEPING PARENTING REAL
COMMUNITY!

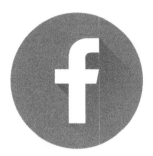

**Join / share our Facebook Group here
(access to all our free books)**

 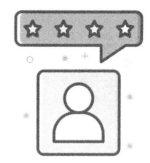

Check out our **Customer Reviews & Testimonials!**

Keeping Parenting Real **Merchandise**and **Full Catalog**

Check out all our product reviews **here**

RECIPES

1. SCRUMPTIOUS SWEET POTATO BEAN TACOS

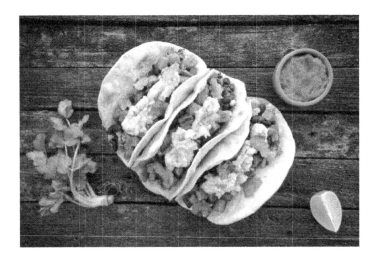

What You'll Need

- Sweet Potato: 5 cups, skinned and minced
- Black Beans: 1 ½ cup, washed and drained
- Corn (frozen): 1 cup, defrost, drained, and brought to room temperature
- Corn Tortillas: 7 to 9 small pcs, heated
- Avocado: 1 cup, diced
- Lime Wedges: 7 to 9 pcs
- Feta Cheese (pasteurized): ¾ cup, crushed

- Cilantro Leaved (fresh): ¾ cup
- Olive Oil: 3 ¼ tbsp
- Yellow Onion: 1 tbsp, minced
- Cumin (ground): ¾ tsp
- Garlic: ½ tsp, diced
- Coriander (ground): ½ tsp
- Chile Powder: ¼ tsp
- Salt and Ground Pepper (fresh), to taste

Directions

1. Preheat oven to 435° F
2. Place sweet potatoes on a baking sheet and coat them with olive oil.
3. Season sweet potatoes with chili powder, and salt and pepper to taste.
4. Arrange sweet potato into a single layer.
5. Bake sweet potatoes for 18 minutes. Stir sweet potato halfway through the 18 minutes. Sweet potatoes will be tender.
6. Place the skillet over medium heat and add olive oil (1 tablespoon) Add onion and cook until translucent and soft (5 minutes).
7. Add garlic and saute until golden (1-2 minutes) Don't let the garlic burn.

8. Sprinkle coriander and cumin over the onions and garlic.
9. Add black beans to the pan and combine with seasoned onions and garlic.
10. Warm up the tortillas in the microwave (15 seconds at a time until heated).
11. Fill the tortilla with black beans, corn, cheese, and avocado, and top with cilantro.
12. Squeeze lemon over taco (optional).

Makes 4 servings

Nutrition facts

Amount per serving	
Calories	830
% Daily Value+	
Total Fat 28g	36%
Saturated Fat 7.1g	36%
Cholesterol 17mg	6%
Sodium 259mg	11%
Total Carbohydrate 118.4g	43%
Dietary Fiber 27.3g	97%
Total Sugars 8.7g	
Protein 34.4g	
Vitamin D 0mcg	0%
Calcium 289mg	22%
Iron 9mg	52%
Potassium 2408mg	51%

*The % Daily Value (DV) tells you how much a nutrient in a food serving contributes to a daily diet. 2,000 calorie a day is used for general nutrition

2. SIMPLE KALE, FRUIT & ALMOND SALAD

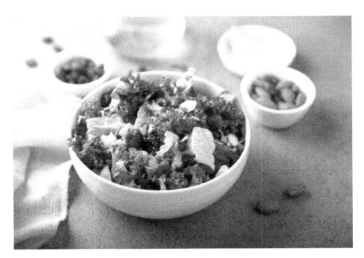

What You'll Need

- Curly Kale: 3 cups
- Cranberries (dried): 1 cup
- Almonds (lightly toasted): 1 ¼ cup, diced
- Figs (dried): ½ cup, minced

Balsamic Vinaigrette

- Olive Oil (extra-virgin): ¾ cup
- Parmesan Cheese: ¾ cup, grated
- Balsamic Vinegar: ½ cup
- Shallot: 1 ¼ tbsp, diced

- Salt and Ground Pepper (fresh), to taste

Directions

1. Rinse and dry kale
2. Prepare the kale by removing tough stems and tearing into small pieces
3. Place kale in the salad bowl and add, figs, cranberries, and almonds, and mix

Balsamic vinaigrette

1. In a small bowl add vinegar, shallots and season with salt and pepper to taste
2. Whisk in olive oil to vinegar mixture
3. Set aside

Salad Prep

1. Slowly add vinaigrette to the kale salad bowl and toss
2. Put aside salad for 12 minutes
3. Add Parmesan to salad and serve

Makes 4 servings

Nutrition facts

Calories	373
	% Daily Value*
Total Fat 32.4g	41%
Saturated Fat 5.1g	25%
Cholesterol 7mg	2%
Sodium 114mg	5%
Total Carbohydrate 15.7g	6%
Dietary Fiber 4.6g	16%
Total Sugars 5.1g	
Protein 9.2g	
Vitamin D 0mcg	0%
Calcium 221mg	17%
Iron 2mg	10%
Potassium 456mg	10%

*The % Daily Value (DV) tells you how much a nutrient in a food serving contributes to a daily diet. 2,000 calorie a day is used for general nu

3. PERFECT COCONUT CHICKEN SPINACH CURRY

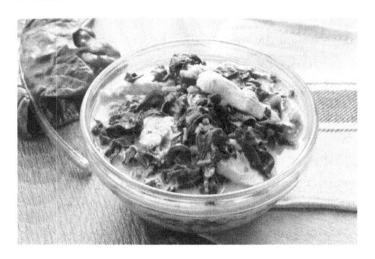

What You'll Need

- Butternut Squash: 1 ¾ cup
- Chicken Breasts (boneless and skinless): 2 ½ cups, chopped
- Coconut Milk: 1 ¾ cup
- Spinach Leaves (fresh): 4 ¼ cup
- Red Bell Pepper: ¼ cup, seeded and chopped
- Yellow Onion: ¼ cup, chopped
- Curry Paste (yellow): 2 ¼ tbsp
- Brown Rice, cooked for serving
- Lime Wedges, to taste

Directions

Butternut squash

1. Preheat the oven to 425° F.
2. Prepare the butternut squash by cutting in half lengthwise and scooping seeds and strings out.
3. Place butternut squash cut side down on a prepared baking sheet.
4. Bake until fork tender (17 minutes).
5. Scoop out the flesh and then dice. Discard the skins

Curry

1. Heat the skillet over medium heat.
2. Open a can of coconut milk and scoop off a thick layer of coconut cream from the top of the can. Add cream to the skillet.
3. Add curry paste to cream and saute for 2 minutes.
4. Add onion, and bell pepper and cook until tender.
5. Add the diced squash, chicken, and remaining coconut milk.

6. Add 10 fl. oz of water to the skillet and stir together with the mixture.

7. Turn up the heat to medium-high, bring the mixture to a boil and reduce heat to medium to simmer until the chicken is cooked (18 minutes).

8. Add Spinach leaves to the mixture and stir to incorporate.

9. Spoon curry over rice

Makes 4 servings

Nutrition facts

Calories	373
	% Daily Value*
Total Fat 32.4g	41%
Saturated Fat 5.1g	25%
Cholesterol 7mg	2%
Sodium 114mg	5%
Total Carbohydrate 15.7g	6%
Dietary Fiber 4.6g	16%
Total Sugars 5.1g	
Protein 9.2g	
Vitamin D 0mcg	0%
Calcium 221mg	17%
Iron 2mg	10%
Potassium 456mg	10%

*The % Daily Value (DV) tells you how much a nutrient in a food serving contributes to a daily diet. 2,000 calorie a day is used for general nu

4. HERBY SKILLET-SEARED SALMON

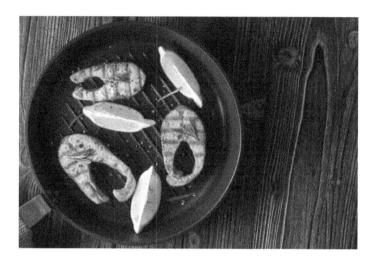

What You'll Need

- Wild Salmon Fillets: 3 to 5 pcs of 180g to 190g, skinned
- French Lentils (green): 3 ¼ cup
- Chicken Stock: 2 ¾ cup
- Leek (white and pale green parts only): 1 ¾ cups, minced
- Carrot: 1 cup, skinned and minced
- Celery (stalk): 1 cup. minced
- Thyme (fresh): 3 to 4 pcs of sprigs
- Italian Parsley (fresh): 2 ¼ sprigs, 1 ¼ tbsp minced, plus more for toppings

- Bay Leaf (dried): ¾ pc
- Olive Oil: 2 ¼ tbsp, plus more for rubbing
- Red Wine Vinegar: 1 ¼ tbsp
- Chives (fresh): 2 ¼ tsp, diced, plus more for toppings
- Tomato Paste: 1 ¼ tbsp
- Garlic: ½ tsp, diced
- Salt and Ground Pepper (fresh), to taste

Directions

1. Soak lentils - pour boiling water over them and let them stand for 15 minutes and then drain the water.
2. Place the skillet over medium-low heat and add 2 tablespoons of olive oil.
3. Saute leeks until tender and brown (8 minutes).
4. Saute garlic for 3 minutes.
5. Add to skillet chicken stock, lentils, celery, carrot, tomato paste, thyme, parsley sprigs, and bay leaf. Stir together.
6. Lower heat and simmer the mixture until your lentils are cooked (23 minutes).

Salmon

1. Preheat the oven to 450° F.
2. Use an oven-proof saute pan and heat over medium heat.
3. Take out salmon and rub olive oil on both sides.
4. Apply salt and pepper to taste over salmon.
5. Put salmon in a heated saute pan and cook. Don't move the salmon on the pan but cook for 3 minutes.
6. With care, flip salmon over and cook for further 3 minutes.
7. Place salmon in the oven and bake until medium-well (7 minutes).

Prepare Salmon and Lentils

1. Remove bay leaf, and herb sprigs from the lentil mixture.
2. Add vinegar, parsley and chives stir.
3. Season salt and pepper to taste.
4. On the serving plate, spoon lentils onto the plate and then top with salmon

Makes 4 servings

Nutrition Facts

Calories	397
	% Daily Value*
Total Fat 11.4g	15%
Saturated Fat 1.7g	8%
Cholesterol 75mg	25%
Sodium 604mg	26%
Total Carbohydrate 31.3g	11%
Dietary Fiber 12.1g	43%
Total Sugars 4.2g	
Protein 43.5g	
Vitamin D 0mcg	0%
Calcium 129mg	10%
Iron 5mg	28%
Potassium 1152mg	25%

*The % Daily Value (DV) tells you how much a nutrient in a food serving contributes to a daily diet. 2,000 calorie a day is used for general nutrition advice.

5. QUICK & EASY STIR-FRIED TOFU & MIXED VEGGIES

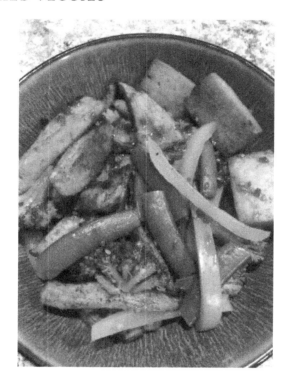

What You'll Need

- Tofu (extra-firm) 1 ¾ cup, sliced
- Sugar Snap Peas: 2 ¼ cup
- Broccoli Florets (small): 2 ¼ cup
- Almonds (lightly toasted): ¾ cup, chopped
- Soy Sauce (low-sodium): 3 ¼ tbsp

- Rice Vinegar: 2 ¼ tbsp
- Vegetable Oil: 2 ¼ tbsp
- Cornstarch: 1 ¼ tbsp
- Ginger (fresh): 1 ¼ tsp, skinned and grated
- Garlic: 1 ¼ tsp, diced
- Brown Rice or Whole Grain Noodles, cooked for serving

Directions

Tofu preparation

1. Drain the water of the tofu from the package.
2. Dry tofu with paper towels.

Optional: prepare a baking sheet with paper towels and put tofu on there (slice so you can distribute tofu in a single layer). Cover the tofu with additional paper towels. Then cover with another baking sheet and weigh down with canned goods and have it drain for 20 minutes)

Stir-fry sauce

1. Whisk together soy sauce, rice vinegar, ginger, garlic, and cornstarch in a medium bowl.

Tofu

1. Heat a wok or a large frying pan over medium heat.
2. Add oil and let it coat the bottom of the pan.
3. Add tofu in a single layer so that it can cook without stirring. Cook until tofu is golden brown (10 minutes).
4. Carefully flip tofu and cook without stirring (8 minutes).
5. When the tofu is done, take it out of the wok or pan and place it on a plate.

Final cooking phase

1. Using the same wok or pan, place it back onto medium heat.
2. Add 6 fl. oz. of water to the pan.
3. Add sugar snap peas and broccoli to the pan and let the water come to a boil. Cover the

pan and let veggies cook until tender-crisp (3 minutes approx). Remove cover.

4. When veggies are tender-crisp add stir-fry sauce and cook until the sauce becomes thick (2 minutes).
5. Add tofu to the pan and coat with sauce.
6. Place rice or noodles on a plate and then top with the stir fry mixture.
7. Add almonds and serve.

Makes 4 servings

Nutrition facts

Nutrition Facts
Servings: 4

Amount per serving

Calories	129

	% Daily Value*
Total Fat 5g	6%
Saturated Fat 1g	5%
Cholesterol 0mg	0%
Sodium 46mg	2%
Total Carbohydrate 12.2g	4%
Dietary Fiber 4.3g	15%
Total Sugars 6.1g	
Protein 12g	
Vitamin D 0mcg	0%
Calcium 274mg	21%
Iron 3mg	17%
Potassium 509mg	11%

*The % Daily Value (DV) tells you how much a nutrient in a food serving contributes to a daily diet. 2,000 calorie a day is used for

6. PAN-SEARED CAULIFLOWER STEAKS WITH HERBED DRESSING

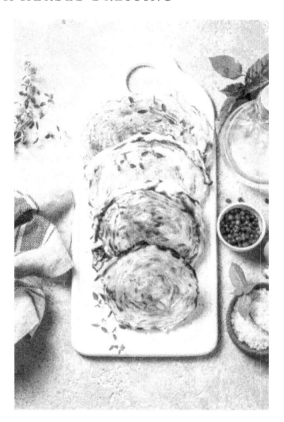

What You'll Need

- Cauliflower (head) 1 to 2 pcs
- Greek Yogurt: ¾ cup
- Olive Oil: 4 ¼ tbsp

- Herbed yogurt
- Italian Parsley (fresh): 2 ¼ tsp, diced
- Lemon Juice (fresh): 1 ¾ tsp
- Coriander (ground): ¾ tsp
- Cumin (ground): ¾ tsp
- Turmeric (ground): ¾ tsp
- Garlic: ½ tsp, diced
- Lemon Zest (grated): ¼ tsp
- Salt (to taste)

Directions

1. Preheat the oven to 435° F.
2. Prepare the cauliflower by removing the tough outer leaves and trim the stem so that the cauliflower can stand upright.
3. Cut four 1/2 inch slices from the center of the cauliflower. Keep the stems on so that the cauliflower won't fall apart.

Herbed yogurt

1. In a medium bowl, mix the yogurt, lemon zest, juice, parsley, garlic, and salt to taste.
2. In a separate small bowl mix the turmeric, cumin, and coriander.

Cauliflower steaks

1. Using a heavy bottom skillet, heat over medium-high heat and add two tablespoons of olive oil, and make sure to coat the bottom of the pan.
2. Sear cauliflower slices (steaks) two at a time in a skillet. Turn once so that you can brown both sides (3 minutes per side).
3. Remove cauliflower slices (steaks) to a baking pan and cook the remaining slices (steaks).
4. When done cooking cauliflower, distribute the spice mixture over the cauliflower. You can rub the spice mixture on the cauliflower to coat it evenly.
5. Season with salt to taste.
6. Bake the cauliflower for 15 minutes.
7. Serve cauliflower right away and top with the herbed yogurt.

Makes 4 servings

Nutrition facts

Nutrition Facts	
Servings: 4	
Amount per serving	
Calories	**129**
	% Daily Value*
Total Fat 5g	6%
Saturated Fat 1g	5%
Cholesterol 0mg	0%
Sodium 46mg	2%
Total Carbohydrate 12.2g	4%
Dietary Fiber 4.3g	15%
Total Sugars 6.1g	
Protein 12g	
Vitamin D 0mcg	0%
Calcium 274mg	21%
Iron 3mg	17%
Potassium 509mg	11%

*The % Daily Value (DV) tells you how much a nutrient in a food serving contributes to a daily diet. 2,000 calorie a day is used for

7. TENDER STEAK FAJITAS

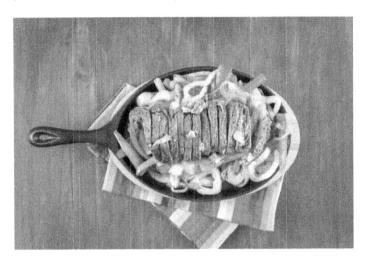

What You'll Need

- Flank Steak: 1x 650g to 750g
- Tortillas (large): 7 to 8 pcs, heated
- Yellow Onion (small): ½ cup, chopped
- Red Bell Pepper (small): ½ cup, seeded and chopped
- Lime Juice: ½ cup
- Avocado: 1 to 3 pcs
- Olive Oil: 2 ¼ tbsp
- Garlic: ½ tsp, diced

For the marinade:

- Lime Juice (fresh): ½ cup
- Cilantro (fresh): ½ cup, diced
- Olive Oil: 1 tbsp
- Jalapeño Pepper: 1 ¼ tsp, diced
- Garlic: 1 ¼ tsp, diced
- Cumin (ground): ¾ tsp
- Salt and Ground Pepper (fresh) to taste

Directions

Marinade

1. Using a gallon zip-lock bag, add lime juice, cilantro, olive oil, jalapeno, garlic, cumin, and salt and pepper (to taste).
2. Add the steak and make sure it gets coated with the marinade.
3. Zip/close the bag and place it in the refrigerator to marinate for no less than one hour. Best if left overnight.

Avocado Mix

1. Scoop the flesh out of the avocado and place it in a medium-sized bowl.
2. Add garlic and lime juice.
3. Using a fork, mash everything together. Leave some chunks.
4. Press plastic wrap on the surface and then seal onto the bowl and refrigerate.

Fajitas

1. Preheat the gas grill (or charcoal) to medium-high heat.
2. Heat olive oil in a skillet over medium-high heat.
3. Add onion and cook until tender (4 minutes) Remove from pan.
4. Add the bell pepper and cook until tender (4 minutes) removed from the pan.
5. Put onion and bell pepper aside (keep warm).
6. Remove steak from marinade.
7. Place steak on a preheated grill and cook until 145F internal temperature (you can flip the steak over and cook according to your preference).

8. Take the steak out to rest for 4 minutes.
9. Slice steak against the grain into thin slices.
10. Warm tortillas.
11. Take out the avocado mixture from the fridge.
12. Place fajita steak slices into a taco and top with avocado mixture.
13. Serve immediately.

Makes 4 servings

Nutrition facts

Nutrition Facts
Servings: 4

Amount per serving

Calories	545
	% Daily Value*
Total Fat 24.9g	**32%**
Saturated Fat 7.9g	**40%**
Cholesterol 90mg	**30%**
Sodium 118mg	**5%**
Total Carbohydrate 30.6g	**11%**
Dietary Fiber 7.4g	**26%**
Total Sugars 3.3g	
Protein 49.9g	
Vitamin D 0mcg	0%
Calcium 78mg	6%
Iron 4mg	23%
Potassium 983mg	21%

*The % Daily Value (DV) tells you how much a nutrient in a food serving contributes to a daily diet. 2,000 calorie a day is used for general nutrition advice.

8. WEEKEND SWISS CHARD & FETA FRITTATA

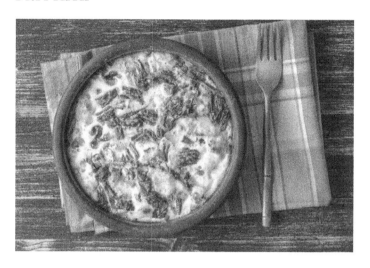

What You'll Need

- Swiss Chard: 3 cups
- Bacon (turkey): 2 to 4 slices, diced
- Eggs (large): 7 to 9 pcs
- Feta Chees (pasteurized): 1 ¼ cup, crushed
- Milk: 1 cup
- Sweet Onion: ½ cup, finely chopped
- Shallot: ¼ cup, diced
- Olive Oil: 1 ¼ tbsp
- Salt and Ground Pepper (fresh) to taste

Directions

1. Preheat the oven to 400° F.
2. Prepare an 8" by 8" baking dish with butter or butter spray*.
3. Cook turkey bacon according to package instructions, and set aside.
4. Heat a small frying pan to medium heat and add olive oil.
5. Add onion and cook until tender (10 minutes).
6. In a medium bowl, crack eggs and whisk until blended - don't over whisk.
7. Add milk and cheese to eggs.
8. Rinse chard and cut out tough stems and chop leaves roughly to make 2 cups.
9. Add shallot to the frying pan and cook for 2 minutes.
10. Add chard to the frying pan with onions and shallot. Cook for 2 minutes or just until the chard is wilted. Stirring gently.
11. Season mixture with salt and pepper to taste.
12. Add frying pan mixture and turkey bacon to the bowl with the eggs and pour the mixture into your prepared baking dish.

13. Bake until the egg mixture is fluffy and golden, (21 minutes).
14. Serve immediately.

*ceramic or glass pan preferred.

Makes 4 servings

Nutrition facts

Nutrition Facts
Servings: 4

Amount per serving

Calories	545

	% Daily Value*
Total Fat 24.9g	32%
Saturated Fat 7.9g	40%
Cholesterol 90mg	30%
Sodium 118mg	5%
Total Carbohydrate 30.6g	11%
Dietary Fiber 7.4g	26%
Total Sugars 3.3g	
Protein 49.9g	
Vitamin D 0mcg	0%
Calcium 78mg	6%
Iron 4mg	23%
Potassium 983mg	21%

*The % Daily Value (DV) tells you how much a nutrient in a food serving contributes to a daily diet. 2,000 calorie a day is used for general nutrition advice.

9. SCRUMMY SHRIMP QUINOA SALAD

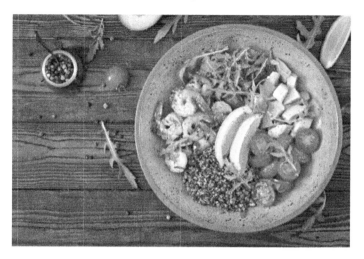

What You'll Need

- Shrimp (medium): ½ kilo, shells removed and deveined
- Avocado: 1 ¼ pc
- Cherry Tomatoes (red or yellow): 1 ¼ cup, sliced in half
- Cilantro Leaves (fresh): 1 ¼ cup
- Quinoa: 1 ¼ cup
- Basil Leaves (fresh): 1 ¼ cup
- Garlic: 1 to 3 pcs, skinned
- Lemon Peel: 1 to 3 strips of 5 cm
- Olive Oil (extra-virgin): 6 ¼ tbsp

- Mint Leaves (fresh): 2 ¼ tbsp
- Green Onions (white and pale green parts only): 1 to 3 pcs, finely chopped
- Salt and Ground Pepper (fresh) to taste

Directions

1. Using a food processor, blend the basil, mint, cilantro, garlic, and lemon peel. Pulse so that the herbs are finely chopped.
2. Place 1 tablespoon of the herb mixture into a medium bowl and add 1 tablespoon of olive oil and salt and pepper to taste.
3. Add shrimp to bowl and coat with herbal mixture.
4. Cover the bowl with plastic wrap and place it in the refrigerator to marinate.
5. Add 4 tablespoons of olive oil to the herb mixture left in the food processor and pulse until the mixture is blended. Transfer to a medium-sized bowl.
6. Add tomato and green onions to the herbal mixture in a bowl. Add salt and pepper to taste and toss to coat. Set aside.

Quinoa

1. In a small saucepan over high heat add quinoa and 1 1/2 cups of water and 1 tablespoon of olive oil.
2. Bring the quinoa mixture to a boil. Reduce heat and cover.
3. Cook for 15-18 minutes until the water is absorbed and the quinoa is tender.
4. Turn off the heat and remove the saucepan. Put aside the saucepan/quinoa to settle for 10 minutes.

Shrimp

1. Take marinating shrimp out of the refrigerator.
2. Remove shrimp from marinade and place on a cooking sheet.
3. Preheat broiler.
4. When the oven is ready, place the shrimp in the oven. Broil for 3-4 minutes until the shrimp is pink and curls into an "O". Be careful not to over broil the shrimp.

Finish

1. Add quinoa to the mixture and toss to coat. Carefully fold in shrimp to the quinoa mixture.
2. Take out the avocado and cut it in half and remove the pit.
3. While avocado is still peeled, slice the flesh into strips horizontally and then vertically. Carefully scoop the flesh out.
4. Add avocado to the mixture and toss to coat.
5. Serve quinoa and shrimp immediately

Makes 4 servings

Nutrition facts

Nutrition Facts

Servings: 4

Amount per serving

Calories	**1557**

	% Daily Value*
Total Fat 46.4g	60%
Saturated Fat 7.3g	37%
Cholesterol 132mg	44%
Sodium 439mg	19%
Total Carbohydrate 256.7g	93%
Dietary Fiber 75.2g	269%
Total Sugars 150g	
Protein 72.2g	
Vitamin D 0mcg	0%
Calcium 672mg	52%
Iron 18mg	102%
Potassium 14154mg	301%

*The % Daily Value (DV) tells you how much a nutrient in a food serving contributes to a daily diet. 2,000 calorie a day is used for general nutrition advice.

10. BREAKFAST OMELETTE STARRING SPINACH & CHEESE

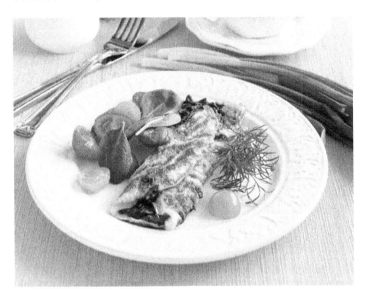

What You'll Need

- Eggs: 1 to 3 pcs
- Swiss Cheese: 1 to 3 slices
- Tomato: ¾ large tomato or 1 ¼ plum tomato, diced
- Spinach: 1 ¼ cup, sliced
- Milk: 3 ¼ tbsp
- Olive Oil (extra-virgin): 1 ¼ tbsp
- Salt and Pepper to taste

Directions

1. In a medium-sized mixing bowl add eggs and milk and beat together until just blended.
2. Add tomatoes and spinach. Season with salt and pepper.
3. In a non-stick skillet over medium heat, add olive oil .
4. Add eggs to skillet and let egg mixture cook for 2 minutes.
5. Add one swiss cheese slice to the left side of the egg mixture.
6. Carefully lift the right side of the eggs and fold over the left side.
7. Place the remaining swiss cheese slice over the omelet and let it melt for 1 minute.
8. Gently remove omelette from the non-skillet and slide it onto the plate.
9. Serve immediately.

Makes 1 serving

Nutrition facts

Nutrition Facts
Servings: 1

Amount per serving

Calories	357

	% Daily Value*
Total Fat 24.6g	31%
Saturated Fat 12.7g	64%
Cholesterol 379mg	126%
Sodium 257mg	11%
Total Carbohydrate 7.2g	3%
Dietary Fiber 1.4g	5%
Total Sugars 3.2g	
Protein 27.6g	
Vitamin D 55mcg	277%
Calcium 526mg	40%
Iron 3mg	15%
Potassium 475mg	10%

*The % Daily Value (DV) tells you how much a nutrient in a food serving contributes to a daily diet. 2,000 calorie a day is used for general nutrition advice.

11. OVEN-BAKED COD & MIXED VEGGIES

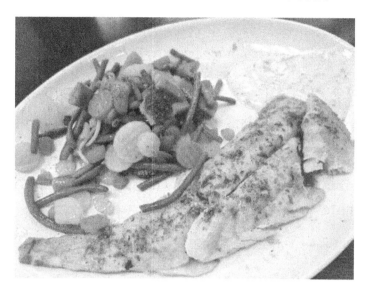

What You'll Need

- Cod Fillets: 1 to 3 pcs of 245g to 255g, sliced in half crosswise
- Asparagus Spears: 7 to 9 pcs, trimmed and chopped diagonally
- Lemon Wedges: 3 to 5 pcs, to serve
- Spinach Leaves: 4 ¼ cup
- Artichoke Hearts: 2 cups, washed and cut lengthwise
- Cherry Tomato: 1 ¼ cup, sliced in half
- Basil (fresh): 2 ¼ tbsp, diced

- Olive Oil: 1 ¼ tbsp
- Chives (fresh): 1 ¼ tbsp, diced
- Capers: 2 ¼ tsp, diced
- Salt and Ground Pepper (fresh) to taste

Directions

1. In a medium-size bowl add asparagus, tomatoes, artichokes, basil, and chives, and drizzle olive oil over the veggies and coat. Add salt and pepper to taste.

2. Preheat the oven to 425° F.

3. Cut off 4 pieces of foil 12 by 20 inches each piece for cooking packets.

4. Prepare each foil packet with the following:

- 1 cup of spinach leaves in the center of the foil piece
- 1 piece of cod over the spinach
- Season packet with salt and pepper
- Add tomato mixture and capers over the cod.

5. Fold the foil packages over the fish and seal the package shut

6. Place foil packages onto a baking sheet and bake for 12 minutes (make sure that the fish is opaque and flakes easily)

7. Transfer the cod mixture to individual plates. Squeeze with lemon if desired.

8. Serve immediately.

Makes 4 servings

Nutrition facts

Nutrition Facts
Servings: 4

Amount per serving

Calories	233

	% Daily Value*
Total Fat 1.6g	2%
Saturated Fat 0.3g	2%
Cholesterol 69mg	23%
Sodium 278mg	12%
Total Carbohydrate 21.8g	8%
Dietary Fiber 11g	39%
Total Sugars 3.9g	
Protein 36.2g	
Vitamin D 0mcg	0%
Calcium 136mg	10%
Iron 5mg	26%
Potassium 1285mg	27%

*The % Daily Value (DV) tells you how much a nutrient in a food serving contributes to a daily diet. 2,000 calorie a day is used for general nutrition advice.

12. HEALTHY & EASY TOFU SESAME SOY SAUCE STIR-FRY

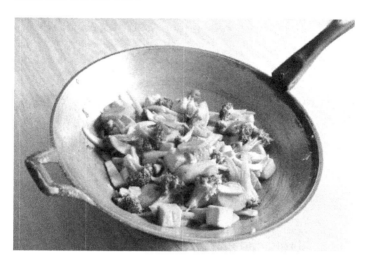

What You'll Need

- Tofu (extra-firm): 2 cups, sliced into cubes
- Green Onions: 2 to 4 pcs, diced
- Water: ½ cup
- Soy Sauce(light): 4 ¼ tbsp
- Vinegar: 2 ¼ tbsp
- Hoisin Sauce: 2 ¼ tbsp
- Chicken Broth: 2 ¼ tbsp
- Ginger: 1 ¼ to 2 ¼ tsp

- Garlic: 1 tsp, diced
- Sesame Oil: ¾ tsp
- Mixed Vegetables (carrots, bell peppers, cabbage, broccoli, snow peas): 4 ¼ cups fresh or 1 ¼ lb frozen

Directions

1. Pat tofu dry with paper towels
2. In a medium-size bowl add sesame oil, soy sauce, vinegar, hoisin sauce, and water and stir together.
3. Add tofu and marinate for 15 minutes

Stir fry

1. Add chicken broth to a nonstick skillet (or wok) and heat (2 minutes).
2. Add garlic and green onion and cook until tender (2 minutes).
3. Add all the vegetables (except for broccoli) and stir-fry until veggies are tender-crisp. (Add chicken broth or water as needed).
4. Add tofu and cook until all sides are brown. Remove tofu from the pan and set it aside.

5. Add broccoli and left-over marinade and stir-fry until broccoli is tender-crisp.
6. Return tofu to the pan and cook until heated (warm).
7. Serve immediately over brown rice.

Makes 4 servings

Nutrition facts

Nutrition Facts
Servings: 4

Amount per serving

Calories	899
	% Daily Value*
Total Fat 17.5g	**22%**
Saturated Fat 2.6g	**13%**
Cholesterol 0mg	**0%**
Sodium 44mg	**2%**
Total Carbohydrate 158.7g	**58%**
Dietary Fiber 12.6g	**45%**
Total Sugars 4.9g	
Protein 29.9g	
Vitamin D 0mcg	0%
Calcium 380mg	29%
Iron 8mg	42%
Potassium 1105mg	24%

The % Daily Value (DV) tells you how much a nutrient in a food serving contributes to a daily diet. 2,000 calorie a day is used for general nutrition advice.

13. TASTY TOFU & MUSHROOM MASSAMAN CURRY

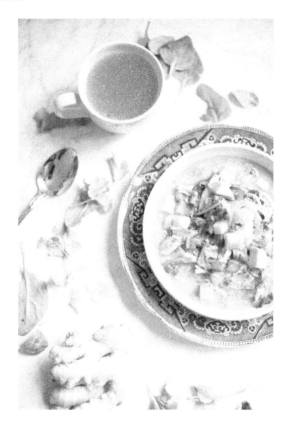

What You'll Need

- Tofu (firm): 1 cup
- Oyster Mushrooms: ¾ cup, slice in half
- Green Beans: ¼ cup, chopped

- Coriander: 5g to 15g, chopped
- Red Bell Pepper: ¼ cup, minced
- The Spice Tailor Thai Massaman Curry: 1x 275g pack
- Vegetable Oil: 2 ½ tbsp
- Breadcrumbs: 2 ½ tbsp
- Salt to taste

Directions

1. Heat 1 tablespoon of oil in a frying pan and saute the mushrooms until they are golden brown on all sides.
2. Season with salt and pepper and cook again for another minute before removing from the pan and setting aside.
3. Heat 1/2 tsp oil in the same pan, add the green beans and stir-fry for 2 minutes.
4. Add the peppers and a pinch of salt, and cook for another two minutes.
5. Place it in a bowl.
6. Blitz the tofu and half of the cooked mushrooms until smooth in a food processor.
7. Chop the remaining mushrooms and combine them with the coriander,

breadcrumbs, and tofu mushroom mix in a mixing bowl.

8. Toss everything together and season to taste.
9. Make 16 walnut-sized balls.
10. Heat the remaining oil in a large frying pan and fry the tofu balls until it turns brown on all sides.
11. Stir-fry for 10 seconds while adding the spices from the spice packet in the pan.
12. Add the massaman paste and coconut sauce and bring to a simmer.
13. Let it simmer for 2-3 minutes after adding the tofu balls.
14. If you plan to eat it with rice, add a little bit of water for a thinner consistency.

Makes 4 servings

Nutrition Facts

Amount per serving
Calories   260

                                    % Daily Value*

Total Fat 9.6g   12%

  Saturated Fat 1.9g   9%

Cholesterol 0mg   0%

Sodium 101mg   4%

Total Carbohydrate 28.2g   10%

  Dietary Fiber 6.2g   22%

  Total Sugars 1.3g

Protein 16.1g

Vitamin D 0mcg   0%

Calcium 129mg   10%

Iron 6mg   33%

Potassium 195mg   4%

*The % Daily Value (DV) tells you how much a
nutrient in a food serving contributes to a daily diet.
2,000 calorie a day is used for general nutrition
advice.

Recipe analyzed by very **well**

14. CHARMING CAULIFLOWER CASHEW CREAM TORTILLAS

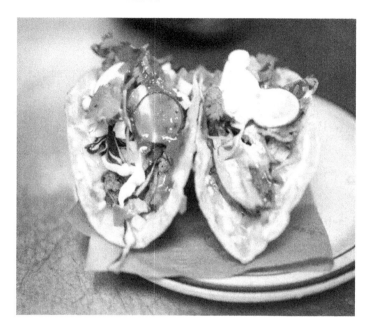

What You'll Need

- Cauliflower: ⅔ of a head
- Purple Cabbage: ½ cup, diced
- Avocado: 1 ½ pc, squashed into quacamole
- Spanish Onion: ½ cup, chopped
- Olive Oil: 1 ½ tbsp
- Water: 1 ¼ tbsp.
- Chilli powder: 2 ½ tsp

- Cumin Powder: 1 ¼ tsp
- Onion Powder: ¾ tsp
- Garlic Powder: ¾ tsp
- Paprika: ¾ tsp
- Coriander Seeds: ¼ tsp, ground
- Tortillas: 8-10 pcs
- Salt and Pepper (to taste)
- Pickled Jalapeños (to taste)
- Lime Wedges (to taste)
- Fresh Herbs (to taste)

Cashew Gravy

- Cashew Nuts: ¾ cup, minced
- Lemon Juice: 1 ¼ tbsp
- Nutritional Yeast: 1 ¼ tbsp
- Water: ½ cup

Directions

1. Preheat the oven to 180°C.
2. Wash the cauliflower and cut them into florets.
3. Combine the garlic powder, onion powder, chili powder, cumin, salt, pepper, and olive oil in a mixing bowl.

4. Add the cauliflower to the spices and spread it out on a baking tray coated with parchment paper.

5. Bake for 30-35 minutes, or until the cauliflower is cooked, stirring halfway through.

6. Make the cashew sauce by putting the cashews in a glass measuring cup and adding enough boiling water to cover the nuts while the cauliflower is cooking. Soak for 20-30 minutes, or until tender.

7. Strain the cashews and combine with the lemon juice and water in a high-powered blender, then set aside.

8. Thinly slice the cabbage, avocado (or mash it), and Spanish onion before serving while the Lime should be cut into wedges.

9. Heat the tortillas as directed on the packet.

10. Place the cauliflower in the center of a tortilla, then layer on the cabbage, avocado, onion, cashew sauce, pickled jalapeños, lime juice, and fresh herbs.

Makes 4 servings

Nutrition Facts

Amount per serving

Calories 305

% Daily Value*

Total Fat 22.2g	**28%**
Saturated Fat 4.3g	**21%**
Cholesterol 0mg	**0%**
Sodium 51mg	**2%**
Total Carbohydrate 24g	**9%**
Dietary Fiber 9.3g	**33%**
Total Sugars 5.2g	
Protein 8.2g	
Vitamin D 0mcg	0%
Calcium 61mg	5%
Iron 3mg	16%
Potassium 845mg	18%

*The % Daily Value (DV) tells you how much a nutrient in a food serving contributes to a daily diet. 2,000 calorie a day is used for general nutrition advice.

15. MOUTH-WATERING PUMPKIN PESTO CHICKEN

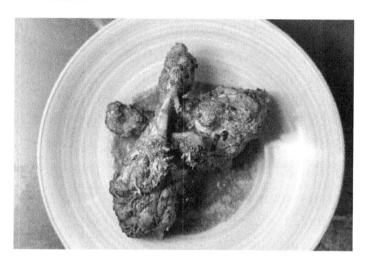

What You'll Need

- Chicken Breasts or Drumsticks: 745g to 755g, boneless and skinless
- Pepitas (hulled green pumpkin seeds): ¾ cup
- Italian Parsley Leaves: 1 ¾ cup
- Cilantro Leaves (fresh): ¾ cup
- Olive Oil: 2 ¼ tbsp plus ¾ cup
- Green Onions: 3 to 5, roughly diced
- Garlic: 1 to 2 cloves, skinned
- Fresh Lemon Juice: 1 ¼ tbsp
- Salt and Pepper (to taste)

Directions

1. Warm 2 tablespoons of olive oil in a frying pan over medium heat.
2. Add the salt, ground pepper, and pepitas, stirring frequently, for 3 to 4 minutes, or until the seeds puff, and turn golden. Set aside to cool.
3. Minced the garlic using a food processor.
4. Combine the parsley, cilantro, green onions, and lemon juice.
5. Take 1/4 cup (2 oz/60 g) of the parsley mixture out of the processor and set it aside.
6. In a zippered plastic bag, place 1/4 cup parsley mixture.
7. Mix in 1/4 cup (2 fl oz/60 ml) olive oil and 1/8 teaspoon pepper into the bag.
8. Add the chicken breasts or drumsticks to the bag, seal it, and massage the chicken to evenly coat it in the marinade. Refrigerate for at least an hour ot upto a day.
9. Add the pumpkin seeds that were set aside to the remaining parsley mixture in the food processor. Pulse until the ingredients are coarsely chopped.
10. Pour the remaining 1/4 cup (2 fl oz/60 ml)

oil and 1/4 cup water into the food processor and mix to a coarse puree.

11. Set aside in a serving bowl.
12. Preheat the grill, whether it's charcoal or gas, to medium-high.
13. Take the chicken out of the marinade and place it on the hottest portion of the grill.
14. Cook for 6 to 8 minutes per side or until well browned on the outside and opaque throughout.
15. After the chicken is cooked, place it on a serving plate and sprinkle it with pesto. Serve while it's hot.

Makes 4 servings

Nutrition Facts

Amount per serving
Calories   704

% Daily Value*

Total Fat 50.5g	65%
Saturated Fat 9.4g	47%
Cholesterol 167mg	56%
Sodium 756mg	33%
Total Carbohydrate 5.2g	2%
Dietary Fiber 1.6g	6%
Total Sugars 0.7g	
Protein 58.7g	
Vitamin D 0mcg	0%
Calcium 67mg	5%
Iron 6mg	31%
Potassium 705mg	15%

*The % Daily Value (DV) tells you how much a nutrient in a food serving contributes to a daily diet. 2,000 calorie a day is used for general nutrition advice.

16. ZEALOUS ZUCCHINI GARLIC SOY NOODLES

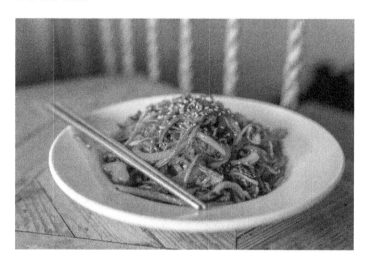

What You'll Need

- Zucchini: 2 to 4 small pcs.

Gravy

- Sesame Oil (toasted): 3 ¼ tbsp
- Soy Sauce (low-sodium): 3 ¼ tbsp
- Garlic: 1 to 3 cloves, diced
- Rice Vinegar: 2 ¼ tbsp
- Peanut Butter: 2 ¼ tbsp
- Tahini: 2 ¼ tbsp

- Sugar: 1 ¼ tbsp
- Chile-Garlic Sauce: 1 ¼ tsp
- Ginger (fresh): ¾ tsp, peeled and grated
- Whole-wheat Spaghetti Pasta: 240g to 260g

Directions

1. Thinly slice the zucchini lengthwise into strips using a mandoline or a very sharp knife, avoiding the seeds in the central portion. Remove the zucchini strips and place them in a separate bowl.
2. Over high heat, bring a pot of salted water to a boil.
3. Prepare the sesame sauce while the water heats up: combine the sesame oil, soy sauce, tahini, peanut butter, vinegar, sugar, chile-garlic sauce, garlic, and ginger in a mixing bowl. Then, set aside.
4. When the water comes to a boil, add the pasta and cook for 7 minutes or until cooked, depending on the package instructions.
5. Scoop out and set aside about 14 cups (2 fl oz/60 ml) of the cooking liquid.

6. Add the zucchini into the pasta and drain them in a colander right after.

7. Transfer to a serving bowl after a quick rinse with cold water.

8. To loosen the sesame sauce, whisk in 1 tablespoon of the cooking liquid, then pour it over the pasta.

9. Toss to coat adding more liquid if needed to reach desired consistency.

10. Place the noodles into a serving bowl and serve while it's hot.

Makes 4 servings

Nutrition Facts

Amount per serving

Calories 399

% Daily Value*

Total Fat 19.9g | **25%**

Saturated Fat 3.1g | **16%**

Cholesterol 46mg | **15%**

Sodium 731mg | **32%**

Total Carbohydrate 44.8g | **16%**

Dietary Fiber 2.2g | **8%**

Total Sugars 6.1g

Protein 12.3g

Vitamin D 0mcg | 0%

Calcium 58mg | 4%

Iron 4mg | 22%

Potassium 436mg | 9%

*The % Daily Value (DV) tells you how much a nutrient in a food serving contributes to a daily diet. 2,000 calorie a day is used for general nutrition advice.

17. PROTEIN-PACKED CHICKEN & BEAN SOUP

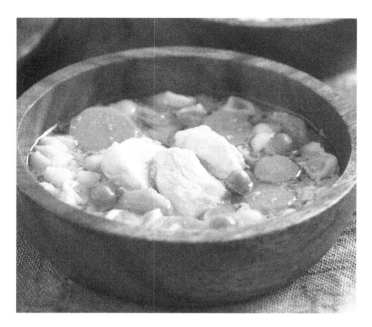

What You'll Need

- Farro (semi-pearled): 1 cup
- Shiitake Mushrooms: 1 cup, cut into slices
- Chicken Breasts or Thighs: ½ kilo, cooked and cut into shreds
- Cannellini Beans: 420g to 430g, washed and drained
- Chicken Stock: 6 ¼ cup

- Carrots: 2 ¼ small pcs, skinned and cut into slices
- Olive Oil: 1 ¼ tbsp
- Italian Parsley (fresh): 1 ¼ tbsp, minced
- Yellow Onion: 1 ¼ small pc, chopped
- Bay Leaf (dried): 1 to 3 pcs
- Thyme Leaves (fresh): 1 ¼ tsp
- Salt and Ground Pepper (to taste)

Directions

1. Warm the olive oil in a Dutch oven over medium-high heat.
2. Sauté the mushrooms for 5 minutes or until they release moisture and start to turn brown. Transfer to a plate and set aside.
3. Next, sauté the onion in a pan for 3 minutes or until it is soft but not browned over medium heat.
4. Add and sauté the carrots for 2 minutes.
5. Add the farro, thyme, and bay leaf to 6 cups of chicken stock.
6. Bring the water to a boil over medium-high heat.
7. Cover the pan and reduce the heat to low and simmer for about 25 minutes or

according to package instructions until the farro is tender.

8. Add the chicken, beans, and mushroom. Simmer until they are cooked thoroughly.
9. If desired, add more stock to thin out the consistency.
10. Make sure to remove and discard the bay leaf.
11. Add the parsley and season it with salt and ground pepper.
12. Transfer it to a bowl and serve while it's hot.

Makes 4 to 6 servings

Nutrition Facts

Amount per serving

Calories 517

% Daily Value*

Total Fat 9.7g	**12%**
Saturated Fat 2.1g	**11%**
Cholesterol 67mg	**22%**
Sodium 1091mg	**47%**
Total Carbohydrate 64.7g	**24%**
Dietary Fiber 20.3g	**73%**
Total Sugars 4.6g	
Protein 43.4g	
Vitamin D 0mcg	0%
Calcium 152mg	12%
Iron 7mg	41%
Potassium 1289mg	27%

*The % Daily Value (DV) tells you how much a nutrient in a food serving contributes to a daily diet. 2,000 calorie a day is used for general nutrition advice.

18. TEMPTING TUNA & BROCCOLI PASTA BAKE

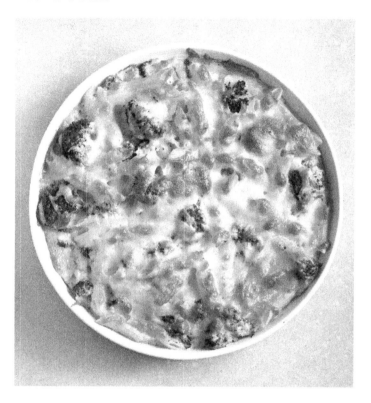

What You'll Need

- Dried Short Pasta (fusilli or penne): 3 cups
- Broccoli Florets (fresh or frozen): 3 ½ cups
- Milk (semi-skimmed): 2 ½ cups

- Tuna (canned): 1 ¼ cup, in water or brine, drained
- Flour (plain): ⅓ cup
- Cheddar (mature): ¼ cup
- Tomato: ¼ cup, chopped (optional)
- Butter: 2 ¾ tbsp
- Salt and Ground Black Pepper (fresh), to taste

Directions

1. Fill a big saucepan halfway with water and bring to boil. Add pasta and cook it according to the package instructions. Add frozen broccoli florets to the pan right before the pasta is cooked and simmer for another 2-3 minutes alongside the pasta.

2. Meanwhile, in a saucepan, boil the butter, flour, and milk over medium heat, whisking continually with a balloon whisk until smooth and thickened to a roux.

3. Continue to cook it, stirring frequently, for another 2-3 minutes, or until the roux has thickened enough to coat the back of a spoon. Add half of the cheese and stir until

melted, then season with salt and freshly ground black pepper to taste.

4. Set the grill's temperature to a maximum and preheat it.

5. In a large colander, drain the pasta and broccoli and transfer it to a shallow ovenproof dish that has been pre-warmed. Shred the tuna on top of the pasta and broccoli.

6. Ladle the cheese sauce on top of the pasta and if desired, garnish it with sliced tomatoes. Then pour the remaining cheese sauce on top of it.

7. Bake the pasta under a high grill for 4 to 5 minutes, or until the cheese begins to melt and turn golden brown. Serve right away.

Makes 4 servings

Nutrition Facts

Nutrition Facts

Servings: 4

Amount per serving

Calories 407

	% Daily Value*
Total Fat 13.1g	17%
Saturated Fat 7.4g	37%
Cholesterol 71mg	24%
Sodium 250mg	11%
Total Carbohydrate 48.7g	18%
Dietary Fiber 2.5g	9%
Total Sugars 8.6g	
Protein 15.9g	
Vitamin D 6mcg	31%
Calcium 261mg	20%
Iron 3mg	16%
Potassium 474mg	10%

*The % Daily Value (DV) tells you how much a nutrient in a food serving contributes to a daily diet. 2,000 calorie a day is used for general nutrition advice.

19. MOREISH PARMESAN PASTA WITH SPINACH & FUNGI

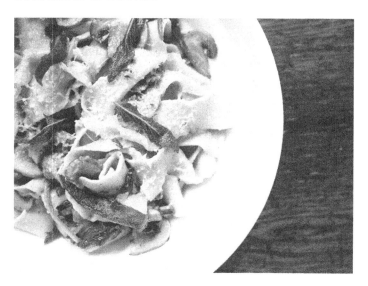

What You'll Need

- Whole-wheat Spaghetti or Bucatini: 225g
- Cremini Mushrooms (fresh): 5 cups, cut into slices
- Baby Spinach (fresh): 4 ¼ cup
- Parmesan Cheese: ½ cup, shredded
- Garlic: 3 to 4 pcs, diced
- Olive Oil (extra virgin): 3 ¼ tbsp
- Lemon Juice: 2 ¼ tbsp
- White Miso: 2 ¼ tbsp

Directions

1. Boil some water in a large pot and cook the pasta according to package instructions.
2. Drain the pasta in a colander and save 1 cup of the cooking water. Set aside.
3. In a large skillet, heat the oil over medium-high heat.
4. Add the mushrooms and garlic and simmer for about 8 minutes or until the mushrooms are soft and start to turn brown while stirring occasionally.
5. In a small mixing bowl, combine half-and-half, miso, and 3/4 cup of the pasta cooking water.
6. Reduce the heat to medium-low and add the half-and-half mixture into the mushroom mixture.
7. Stir it continuously for about a minute or until the miso breaks down.
8. Add the spinach and the parmesan cheese while stirring it constantly for about 2 minutes or until it slightly thickens and the spinach wilts.
9. Add the pasta and gently toss it to coat evenly. If needed, you may add more

cooking water to achieve desired consistency.

10. Remove the pan from the heat and mix in the lemon juice before serving.

Makes 4 servings

Nutrition Facts

Amount per serving
Calories   435

% Daily Value*

Total Fat 18g   23%

  Saturated Fat 5g   25%

Cholesterol 67mg   22%

Sodium 514mg   22%

Total Carbohydrate 52.9g   19%

  Dietary Fiber 4g   14%

  Total Sugars 3.3g

Protein 18.5g

Vitamin D 0mcg   0%

Calcium 250mg   19%

Iron 7mg   37%

Potassium 1425mg   30%

*The % Daily Value (DV) tells you how much a
nutrient in a food serving contributes to a daily diet.
2,000 calorie a day is used for general nutrition
advice.

20. DELISH VEG-CHICK QUESADILLAS

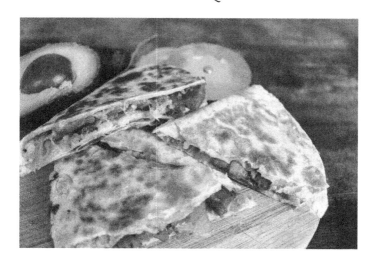

What You'll Need

- Whole Wheat Tortilla: 1x 8 to 10-inch diameter
- Chicken: ½ cup, cooked and cut into shreds
- Cheese: 3 ¼ tbsp, grated
- Corn Kernels: 2 ¼ tbsp, fresh or frozen
- Canola Oil: 2 ¼ tsp
- Onion: ½ cup, diced
- Red Bell Pepper: ½ cup, chopped
- Zucchini: ½ cup, chopped
- Cilantro (fresh): 1 ¼ tbsp (to taste)

Directions

1. In a medium size skillet, heat the oil over medium heat.
2. Add onion, bell pepper, and zucchini and stir them constantly for about 3 to 4 minutes or until the vegetables are tender.
3. Add chicken and corn and cook for about a minute or until they are both heated through.
4. Add the cilantro. (optional)
5. Place the mixed vegetables into a small bowl. Wash the skillet properly before putting it back on the stove.
6. On a cutting board, place the tortilla and sprinkle it with 1 tbsp of cheese leaving a ½ inch border.
7. Add the veggie mixture and the remaining 2 tbsp of cheese and fold the tortilla in half.
8. Over medium heat, cook the quesadilla in a skillet for about 2 minutes per side, or until the tortilla is browned and the cheese has begun to melt.
9. To serve, slice it into three wedges.

Makes 1 serving

Nutrition Facts

Amount per serving

Calories 484

% Daily Value*

Total Fat 16.9g	**22%**
Saturated Fat 3g	**15%**
Cholesterol 50mg	**17%**
Sodium 157mg	**7%**
Total Carbohydrate 64.3g	**23%**
Dietary Fiber 9.8g	**35%**
Total Sugars 13.2g	
Protein 29g	
Vitamin D 0mcg	0%
Calcium 71mg	5%
Iron 9mg	49%
Potassium 1115mg	24%

*The % Daily Value (DV) tells you how much a nutrient in a food serving contributes to a daily diet. 2,000 calorie a day is used for general nutrition advice.

21. CREAMY CHEESE CHICKEN COBB

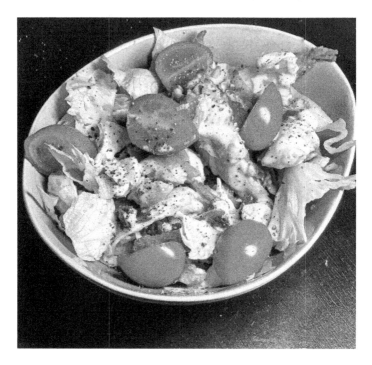

What You'll Need

- Chicken Breast: ⅔ cup, grilled or roasted, cut into cubes or strips
- Romaine Lettuce: 2 ¼ cup
- Cannellini Beans (no salt added): ½ cup, washed and drained
- Tomato: ½ cup, diced
- Hard-boiled Egg: ¾ , diced

- White Button Mushrooms: ½ cup, chopped
- Cucumber: ½ cup, diced
- Blue Cheese Dressing: 2 ¼ tbsp

Directions

1. In a medium-size bowl, place the lettuce.
2. Add 1 tbsp dressing and toss to coat evenly.
3. On top of the lettuce, arrange the tomato, cucumber, mushrooms, chicken, egg, and beans in rows.
4. Sprinkle the remaining 1 tbsp of dressing on top.

Makes 1 serving

Nutrition Facts

Amount per serving
Calories   500

% Daily Value*

Total Fat 20.9g   **27%**

Saturated Fat 3.7g   **19%**

Cholesterol 141mg   **47%**

Sodium 426mg   **19%**

Total Carbohydrate 43.2g   **16%**

Dietary Fiber 15.7g   **56%**

Total Sugars 5.3g

Protein 37.3g

Vitamin D 71mcg   354%

Calcium 132mg   10%

Iron 9mg   51%

Potassium 1512mg   32%

*The % Daily Value (DV) tells you how much a nutrient in a food serving contributes to a daily diet. 2,000 calorie a day is used for general nutrition advice.

22. PUNCHY PUMPKIN CHICKPEA SOUP

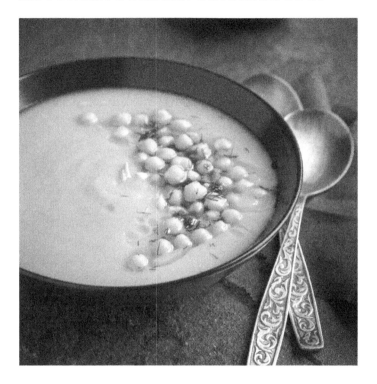

What You'll Need

- Butternut Squash Soup: 425g
- Chickpeas: 1 cup, washed
- Avocado: 2 ¼ tbsp, chopped (optional)
- Greek Yogurt (non-fat): 1 ¼ tbsp
- Lime Juice: 1 ¼ tbsp
- Curry Powder: 1 ¼ tsp

- Salt

Directions

1. In a small saucepan, heat the soup with chickpeas, lime juice, curry powder, and salt.
2. Serve with a dollop of yogurt and a slice of avocado on top.

Makes 1 serving

Nutrition Facts

Amount per serving

Calories 808

% Daily Value*

Total Fat 17.9g	23%
Saturated Fat 1.7g	9%
Cholesterol 0mg	0%
Sodium 784mg	34%
Total Carbohydrate 137g	50%
Dietary Fiber 32.2g	**115%**
Total Sugars 27.3g	
Protein 34.3g	
Vitamin D 0mcg	0%
Calcium 278mg	21%
Iron 12mg	68%
Potassium 1471mg	31%

*The % Daily Value (DV) tells you how much a nutrient in a food serving contributes to a daily diet. 2,000 calorie a day is used for general nutrition advice.

23. SUCCULENT SLOPPY JOES WITH BEANS

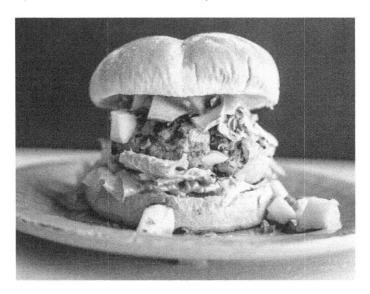

What You'll Need

- Ground Beef (90%-lean): 340g
- Hamburger Buns (whole wheat): 2 to 4 pcs, sliced in half and toasted
- Black Beans (no salt added): 1 ¼ cup, washed
- Onion: 1 ¼ cup, minced
- Tomato Sauce (no-salt-added): 1 ¼ cup
- Ketchup: 3 ¼ tbsp
- Olive Oil (extra virgin): 1 ¼ tbsp
- Worcestershire Sauce (reduced-sodium): 1 ¼ tbsp

- Chile powder: 2 ¼ tsp
- Brown Mustard (spicy): 2 ¼ tsp
- Light Brown Sugar: 1 ¼ tsp
- Garlic Powder: ¾ tsp
- Onion Powder: ¾ tsp
- Cayenne Pepper: 1 pinch

Directions

1. In a large nonstick skillet, heat the oil over medium-high heat.
2. Add beef and cook it for about 3 to 4 minutes or until it turns light brown but not completely cooked through, break it up using a wooden spoon.
3. Transfer the beef to a medium bowl with a slotted spoon, retaining the drippings in the pan.
4. Add the beans and onion to the pan and cook for about 5 minutes or until the onion is softened while stirring it frequently.
5. Add the chile powder, garlic powder, onion powder, and cayenne, and stir for about 30 seconds until you smell the aroma.
6. Add the tomato sauce, ketchup,

Worcestershire, mustard, and brown sugar into the pan.

7. Put back the beef into the pan and let it simmer while stirring it for about 5 minutes or until the beef is cooked and the sauce has thickened slightly.

8. Let it cool down and serve on hamburger buns.

Makes 4 servings

Nutrition Facts

Amount per serving

Calories 479

% Daily Value*

Total Fat 11.3g	14%
Saturated Fat 3g	15%
Cholesterol 76mg	25%
Sodium 821mg	36%
Total Carbohydrate 56.5g	21%
Dietary Fiber 10.9g	39%
Total Sugars 12g	
Protein 39.7g	
Vitamin D 0mcg	0%
Calcium 111mg	9%
Iron 20mg	110%
Potassium 1376mg	29%

*The % Daily Value (DV) tells you how much a nutrient in a food serving contributes to a daily diet. 2,000 calorie a day is used for general nutrition advice.

24. PAN-FRIED LASAGNA, RAVIOLI-STYLE

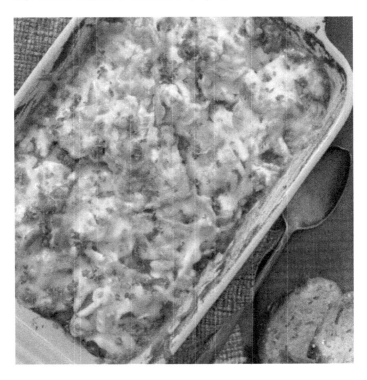

What You'll Need

- Cheese Ravioli: 680g, frozen or refrigerated
- Ground Beef: 2 cups
- Tomatoes (no-salt-added): 3 cups, mashed
- Mozzarella Balls (fresh): 1 cup small size, separated into parts
- Basil (fresh): ½ cup, minced

- Dried Oregano: 1 ¾ tsp
- Garlic Powder: ¾ tsp
- Salt: ¾ tsp
- Ground Pepper: ½ tsp

Directions

1. Preheat the oven.
2. Bring water to a boil in a big pot and cook the ravioli according to package instructions. Drain and set aside.
3. In a large cast-iron or oven-safe pan, sauté ground beef in medium-high heat until cooked for about 4 to 5 minutes while crumbling the beef using the back of the wooden spoon.
4. Add oregano, garlic powder, salt, and pepper to taste.
5. Add basil and tomato and bring to a simmer.
6. Combine and fold the cooked ravioli and half of the mozzarella balls
7. Place the remaining mozzarella balls on top of the pasta.
8. Place the pan in the oven with caution.
9. Broil for 2 to 3 minutes or until the cheese is melted.

Makes 4 servings

Nutrition Facts

Amount per serving

Calories 553

% Daily Value*

Total Fat 20.7g	**27%**
Saturated Fat 9.8g	**49%**
Cholesterol 121mg	**40%**
Sodium 797mg	**35%**
Total Carbohydrate 42.7g	**16%**
Dietary Fiber 10.1g	**36%**
Total Sugars 12g	
Protein 45.4g	
Vitamin D 0mcg	0%
Calcium 297mg	23%
Iron 16mg	90%
Potassium 315mg	7%

*The % Daily Value (DV) tells you how much a nutrient in a food serving contributes to a daily diet. 2,000 calorie a day is used for general nutrition advice.

25. SPICY SMOKED TURKEY & BEANS

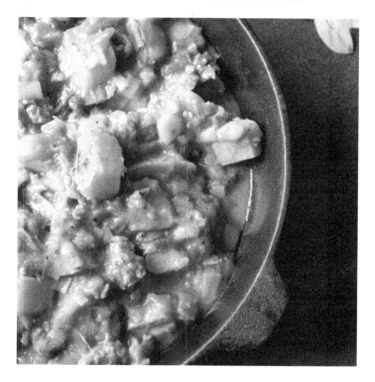

What You'll Need

- Ground Turkey: 2 cups
- Tomatoes (fire-roasted): 1 ¾ cup, minced and undrained
- Black Beans (no-salt-added): 1 ½ cup, washed
- Pumpkin Puree (unseasoned): 2 cups

208 | MEGHAN PARKES

- Kale Leaves (curly): 2 ¼ cups, diced
- Garlic: 4 ½ tsp, diced
- Green Bell Pepper: ¼ cup, diced
- Yellow Onion: 2 cups, diced
- Water: 1 ¾ cup
- Sour Cream: 4 ¼ tbsp
- Chili Powder: 1 ¼ tbsp
- Ground Cumin: 1 ¾ tsp
- Paprika (smoked): 1 ¼ tsp
- Ground Pepper: ½ tsp
- Salt: ¼ tsp
- Fresh Cilantro (fresh), sprinkle on top

Directions

1. In a large saucepan, heat the oil over medium-high heat.
2. Put the onion, garlic, and pepper and stir frequently for about 5 minutes or until the vegetables are tender.
3. Add the turkey and stir for about 5 minutes or until it turns brown.
4. Add beans, beans, water, pumpkin, cumin, chili powder, smoked paprika, pepper, and salt.

5. Bring to a boil, stirring occasionally, over medium-high heat.
6. Reduce the heat to low and cover the pan.
7. Let it simmer while stirring occasionally for about 20 minutes or until the flavors meld.
8. Add the kale during the last 5 minutes of cooking.
9. Pour into 4 bowls and top with 1 spoonful of sour cream in each. You can also serve it with cilantro if desired.

Making 4 servings

Nutrition Facts

Amount per serving

Calories 733

% Daily Value*

Total Fat 21.2g	**27%**
Saturated Fat 4.8g	**24%**
Cholesterol 121mg	**40%**
Sodium 851mg	**37%**
Total Carbohydrate 87.7g	**32%**
Dietary Fiber 22.6g	**81%**
Total Sugars 11.4g	
Protein 57.9g	
Vitamin D 0mcg	0%
Calcium 254mg	20%
Iron 11mg	59%
Potassium 2581mg	55%

*The % Daily Value (DV) tells you how much a nutrient in a food serving contributes to a daily diet. 2,000 calorie a day is used for general nutrition advice.

26. CHEESY CHICKEN SPINACH PASTA

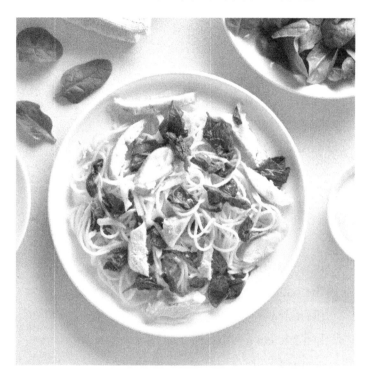

What You'll Need

- Spaghetti Pasta (whole-wheat): 3 cups
- Chicken Breasts: 3 to 5 pcs of 113g, boneless and skinless
- Artichoke Hearts: 1 cup, diced, washed, and squeezed dry
- Baby Spinach: 3 cups, chopped

- Milk (reduced-fat): 1 cup
- Parmesan Cheese: ¾ cup, grated
- Cream Cheese (reduced-fat): ½ cup, sliced into squares
- Olive Oil: 1 ½ tbsp
- Water: 1 ½ tbsp
- Garlic Powder: 1 to 3 tsp
- Kosher Salt: ½ tsp, split into parts
- Ground Pepper: ½ tsp, split into parts

Directions

1. Bring water to a boil in a saucepan. Follow the package guidelines for cooking pasta then drain.
2. Drizzle each chicken with ⅛ tsp salt and pepper.
3. In a skillet, heat the oil over medium heat.
4. Cook the chicken until it turns brown and the instant-read thermometer reads 165°F when inserted into the thickest section. Place on a plate to cool.
5. In a large saucepan, combine spinach and water. Cook them while stirring periodically for about 2 minutes or until they are wilted over medium heat.

6. Put the cream cheese and milk and stir until the cream cheese is melted.
7. Add the garlic powder, parmesan, and the remaining 1/8 teaspoon salt and pepper and whisk it until it's bubbly and thickens.
8. Toss in the artichoke and the cooked pasta and mix.
9. Distribute the pasta mixture into four bowls. Place the thinly sliced chicken breast on top of the spaghetti. If desired, top with more Parmesan cheese.

Making 4 servings.

Nutrition Facts

Amount per serving

Calories 640

% Daily Value*

Total Fat 26.4g	**34%**
Saturated Fat 11.2g	**56%**
Cholesterol 188mg	**63%**
Sodium 591mg	**26%**
Total Carbohydrate 50.5g	**18%**
Dietary Fiber 6.3g	**23%**
Total Sugars 3.9g	
Protein 51.7g	
Vitamin D 24mcg	119%
Calcium 285mg	22%
Iron 6mg	34%
Potassium 1072mg	23%

*The % Daily Value (DV) tells you how much a nutrient in a food serving contributes to a daily diet. 2,000 calorie a day is used for general nutrition advice.

27. JUICY CHICKEN TENDER FAJITAS

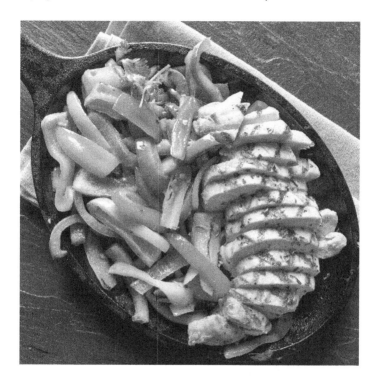

What You'll Need

- Chicken Tenders: 570g
- Black Beans (no-salt-added): 1 ½ cups, washed
- Stemmed Kale: 4 ¼ cups, minced
- Greek Yogurt (plain low-fat): ½ cup
- Yellow Onion: 2 cups, chopped

- Red Bell Pepper: ½ cup, chopped
- Green Bell Pepper: ½ cup, chopped
- Olive Oil: 2 ¼ tbsp, split into parts
- Lime Juice: 1 ¼ tbsp
- Chili Powder: 2 ¼ tsp
- Ground Cumin: 2 ¼ tsp
- Salt: 1 tsp, split into parts
- Garlic Powder: ¾ tsp
- Smoked Paprika: ¾ tsp
- Ground Pepper: ½ tsp
- Water: 2 ¼ tsp

Directions

1. Preheat the oven to 425 degrees F and place a big rimmed baking sheet inside.
2. In a large mixing bowl, combine the salt, garlic powder, paprika, and ground pepper.
3. Set aside ⅓ of the spice mixture in a medium bowl.
4. In the large mixing bowl, whisk 1 tbsp. oil into the remaining mixture.
5. Toss in the chicken, onion, and red and green bell peppers and mix.
6. Take the pan out of the oven and cover it

with cooking spray. Put the chicken mixture evenly and roast it for 15 minutes.

7. Meanwhile, mix the kale and black beans with the remaining 1/4 tsp of salt and 1 tbsp of olive oil and toss to coat in a large mixing basin.

8. Take the pan out of the oven and stir the chicken and vegetables.

9. Distribute the kale and beans evenly on top and roast it for another 5 to 7 minutes or until the chicken is cooked through and the vegetables are tender.

10. Meanwhile, combine the yogurt, lime juice, and water into the set-aside spice mixture to make a yogurt dressing.

11. In four separate bowls, divide the chicken and vegetable mixture. Serve with a yogurt dressing on top.

Making 4 servings.

Nutrition Facts

Amount per serving

Calories 806

% Daily Value*

Total Fat 20g	26%
Saturated Fat 4.6g	23%
Cholesterol 127mg	42%
Sodium 645mg	28%
Total Carbohydrate 88.4g	32%
Dietary Fiber 20.3g	72%
Total Sugars 6.6g	
Protein 71g	
Vitamin D 0mcg	0%
Calcium 371mg	29%
Iron 10mg	58%
Potassium 2787mg	59%

*The % Daily Value (DV) tells you how much a nutrient in a food serving contributes to a daily diet. 2,000 calorie a day is used for general nutrition advice.

28. NOURISHING TURKEY SPINACH CHICKPEA GOULASH

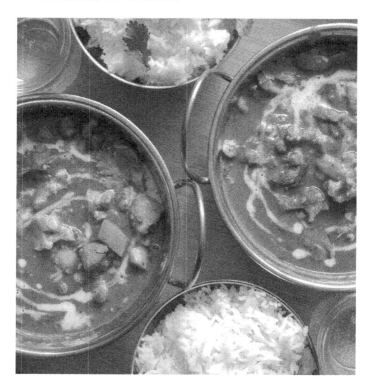

What You'll Need

- Chickpeas: 3 ¾ cup, washed and split into parts
- Ground Turkey (93%-lean): 1 ½ cup
- Chicken Broth (low-sodium): 4 ¼ cup
- Spinach (IQF): 3 ¼ cup

- Onion: 1 ¼ cup diced
- Carrots: 1 cup, chopped
- Garlic: ½ tbsp, diced or ½ tsp, garlic powder
- Tomato Paste: 3 ¼ tbsp
- Olive Oil: 1 ¼ tbsp
- Fennel Seeds: ¾ tsp, crushed
- Red Pepper: ¾ tsp, crushed
- Dried Oregano: ¾ tsp
- Ground Pepper: ½ tsp
- Salt: ¼ tsp
- Parmesan Cheese: ½ cup (to taste)

Directions

1. Using a potato masher or fork, mash 1 can of chickpeas then set it aside.
2. In a big pot, heat the oil over medium-high heat.
3. Add turkey, oregano, fennel seeds, and crushed red pepper and cook them for about 2 to 3 minutes or until the turkey is no longer pink while crushing them with a wooden spoon.
4. Add carrots, onion, and garlic (or garlic powder) and cook for about 3 to 4 minutes,

or until softened and fragrant while stirring often.

5. Add the tomato paste and stir constantly for 30 seconds.

6. In a large pot, combine the broth, mashed and whole chickpeas, pepper, and salt. Cover the pan and let it simmer.

7. Reduce heat to medium-low and cook for about 10 minutes or until the veggies are soft and the flavors have melded.

8. Increase heat to medium-high.

9. Add the spinach and cook it for about 1 to 2 minutes or until the spinach is heated through.

10. Pour the soup into bowls and sprinkle each serving with parmesan if desired.

Making 4 servings.

Nutrition Facts

Amount per serving

Calories   1049

% Daily Value*

Total Fat 27.5g   35%

Saturated Fat 4.4g   22%

Cholesterol 92mg   31%

Sodium 1004mg   44%

Total Carbohydrate 139.5g   51%

Dietary Fiber 39.6g   142%

Total Sugars 27.1g

Protein 70.4g

Vitamin D 0mcg   0%

Calcium 358mg   28%

Iron 17mg   92%

Potassium 2493mg   53%

*The % Daily Value (DV) tells you how much a nutrient in a food serving contributes to a daily diet. 2,000 calorie a day is used for general nutrition advice.

29. HEART-WARMING VEG LENTIL STEW

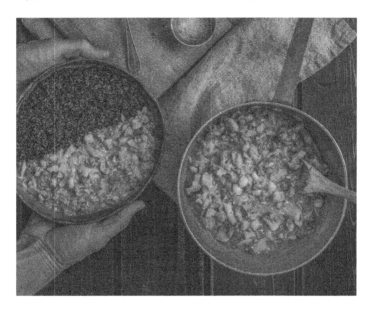

What You'll Need

- Green or Brown Lentils: 1 ¾ cup
- Vegetable or Chicken Broth (low-sodium): 4 ¼ cup
- Mirepoix (mix of chopped onions, carrots, and celery): 3 ¼ cup, fresh or frozen
- Lacinato Kale: 3 ¼ cup, minced
- Tomatoes (unsalted): 2 cup, minced and drained
- Parmesan Cheese: ¾ cup, grated

- Olive Oil (extra-virgin): 2 ¼ tbsp
- Red-wine Vinegar: 1 ¾ tbsp
- Garlic: 4 tsp, chopped
- Thyme (fresh): 2 ¼ tsp, minced
- Ground Pepper: ¾ tsp
- Red Pepper: ¾ tsp, crushed
- Salt: ¾ tsp
- Flat-leaf Parsley (fresh), minced for garnish
- Parmesan Rind (to taste)

Directions

1. In a Dutch oven or large pot, heat the oil over medium heat.
2. Put the onion, carrot, and celery mix and cook for 6 to 10 minutes while stirring occasionally.
3. Add garlic and stir for about 30 seconds or until fragrant.
4. Combine the broth, lentils, tomatoes, thyme, salt, pepper, crushed red pepper, and, if using, the Parmesan rind. On medium-high heat, bring it to a boil.
5. Cover the pot and reduce the heat to low and let it simmer while stirring occasionally for 15 to 25 minutes until lentils are almost

soft, adding water as needed to achieve desired consistency.

6. Add the kale and mix well. Cook for about 5 to 10 minutes or until the kale is soft.
7. If you're using Parmesan rind, remove and discard it.
8. Pour in the vinegar and mix well.
9. To serve, divide the soup into 6 bowls and top with Parmesan cheese. If desired, you can also top it with parsley.

Making 6 servings.

Nutrition Facts

Amount per serving
Calories 278

% Daily Value*

Total Fat 14.8g	19%
Saturated Fat 7g	35%
Cholesterol 30mg	10%
Sodium 1204mg	52%
Total Carbohydrate 15.1g	5%
Dietary Fiber 4.4g	16%
Total Sugars 3.5g	
Protein 19.3g	
Vitamin D 0mcg	0%
Calcium 436mg	34%
Iron 2mg	13%
Potassium 525mg	11%

*The % Daily Value (DV) tells you how much a nutrient in a food serving contributes to a daily diet. 2,000 calorie a day is used for general nutrition advice.

30. AROMATIC CREAMY COCONUT VEG & BEAN CURRY

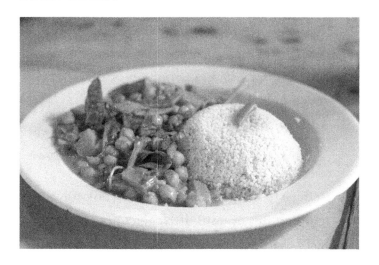

What You'll Need

- Chickpeas: 1 ½ cup, washed and drained
- Coconut Curry Sauce: 1 ¾ cup
- Baby Spinach: 4 ¼ cup
- Onion: 1 ¼ cup, diced
- Zucchini: 1 cup, cut in half and sliced
- Bell Pepper: 1 ¼ cup, chopped
- Vegetable Broth: ¾ cup
- Avocado or Canola Oil: 2 ¼ tsp
- Brown Rice (precooked): 2 ¼ cups, heated according to instructions

Directions

1. In a large skillet, heat the oil over medium-high heat.
2. Add the onion, pepper, and zucchini and cook it for about 5 to 6 minutes or until the zucchini turns brown.
3. Add the chickpeas, simmer sauce, and vegetable broth, and let it simmer while stirring.
4. Reduce to medium-low heat and cook for 4 to 6 minutes or until the veggies are soft.
5. Just before serving, add the spinach and mix well.
6. Serve it over rice.

Making 6 servings.

Nutrition Facts

Amount per serving

Calories 823

	% Daily Value*
Total Fat 9.8g	13%
Saturated Fat 4g	20%
Cholesterol 0mg	0%
Sodium 437mg	19%
Total Carbohydrate 148.9g	54%
Dietary Fiber 24.8g	89%
Total Sugars 16.7g	
Protein 31.1g	
Vitamin D 0mcg	0%
Calcium 198mg	15%
Iron 10mg	57%
Potassium 1612mg	34%

*The % Daily Value (DV) tells you how much a nutrient in a food serving contributes to a daily diet. 2,000 calorie a day is used for general nutrition advice.

BONUS - HEALTHY SNACKS FOR PREGNANCY

(LARGEMAN-ROTH, R.D., 2021)

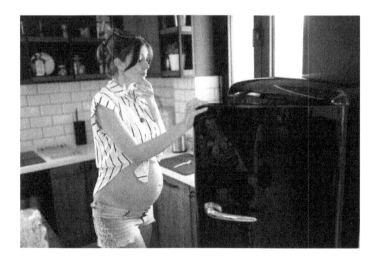

H ere are some ideas for 9 healthy snacks.

1. Egg and English Muffin

You can have your egg scrambled or fried on your muffin. If you don't have any English muffins, wheat toast is a good substitute.

Don't worry about eating the egg yolk as it is a good source of vitamin D and choline.

2. Apple and hard cheese (ex. cheddar, Monterey jack)

This is a great snack for the first trimester as the fiber in the apple can help with your morning sickness.

3. Greek yogurt parfait

Top your parfait with your favorite fruit. Blueberries pack a healthy dose of fiber and an antioxidant boost. Add nuts like walnuts and you get fiber and omega-3 fats. Walnuts in particular have biotin which can be an energy boost.

4. Trail mix

Look for varieties that contain good stuff like pumpkin seeds, almonds, walnuts, unsweetened coconut, cashews, and mango. You can also have dark chocolate as a treat in your trail mix.

5. Avocado toast

Can you believe that avocado can help keep away your leg cramps? It's true, avocado has 345 mg. of potassium. Increasing your potassium intake can help prevent those leg cramps.

6. Veggies and guacamole

Pick your favorite dipping veggies like cucumber and celery and have a fiesta with your homemade guacamole. All it takes is a little lemon juice and maybe a 1/2 teaspoon of jalapeno to brighten up your guacamole dip. Remember that cucumber and celery contain about 96% of water and carrots are 87% water. This is great for boosting your water intake.

7. Cottage cheese and healthy add-ins

Add anything healthy to your cottage cheese and you have a great quick snack. Fruits like strawberries, mango, and apples go well with cottage cheese.

8. Waffles with cashew butter

If you don't like cashew butter, try almond butter or

even natural peanut butter (remember, you want to lower your sugar intake.)

9. Melon and lime

Melons are naturally high in water so eating them can help you with your water intake. Squeeze some lime over it and you have a great snack. Try watermelon or cantaloupe for this snack. Watermelon has 170 mg of potassium!

10. Whole grain tortilla wrap with hummus and tomatoes

Check your store for healthy tortilla wraps. Usually stocked with tortillas, there are different kinds of wrap: whole wheat, vegetable, etc. You can also get creative with the hummus and buy any flavor to your liking. Hummus has both protein and iron.

What other snacks can you think of? A mid-morning snack or an afternoon snack can really help not only with an energy boost but also help to contribute towards your nutrient totals for the day. So snack happy!

FINAL WORDS

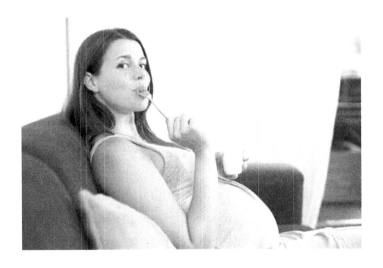

An exciting thing happened to me during my last pregnancy: I maintained a healthy weight! How did I do this? I followed all the advice I received about eating healthy. Before this pregnancy, I ate healthily but I struggled with eating for two.

I had successful pregnancies and healthy babies but for my last pregnancy, I wanted to go out with a bang. Except for this one week when I binged on Mexican sweetbread (what a great week that was!) I stayed away from sugar and did all I could to include all the nutrients in my diet that my baby needed.

Instead of having a 10lb baby, my little girl was a healthy 8lbs. It was a great pregnancy because I felt good all the time. Instead of indulging in donuts, I reached for apples and oranges instead. I learned to include spinach and kale in my salads. Surprisingly, I enjoyed the food choices that I was making and was proud of myself for sticking to a healthy meal plan.

It's a new world of eating healthy for your baby. By making good food choices, you increase your baby's chances of thriving in your womb and being born healthy.

You've learned from this book what to include in your diet and what foods you should avoid. You've learned the specific nutrients you need to consume and exactly why those nutrients are so important.

Then for a little fun, you learned some really healthy recipes to include in your pregnancy meal plan.

Gosh, you should feel fantastic! Now you must be glowing. People are going to start telling you that pregnancy suits you. All because you made some great food choices (and of course, read this book!)

I am so proud of you! You've got everything you need to succeed. Plus, you have our good wishes for a healthy pregnancy and a very healthy baby.

As always, listen to your obstetrician or midwife, they are the ultimate authority on what is good for you during your pregnancy. We hope that this book better equips you to have fruitful conversations about what is right for you during your pregnancy.

Pregnant women come in all shapes and sizes. All pregnant women are a masterpiece in the making. Remember to not get overwhelmed by taking baby steps towards good nutrition. Even when you think you can't eat another vegetable or drink another glass of milk, this book will be there when you need to find healthy alternatives.

Thank you for letting us walk with you during your pregnancy journey. Best of luck! Although you won't need it because: Mommy always knows best!

A FINAL MESSAGE FROM THE AUTHOR:

Reviews are not easy to come by.
As independent authors with a tiny marketing budget,
we rely on readers like you, to leave a short review on Amazon.
Even if it's just a sentence or two!
Simply visit:
Amazon.com/RYP

Customer Reviews

⭐⭐⭐⭐⭐ 2
5.0 out of 5 stars ▾

5 star		100%
4 star		0%
3 star		0%
2 star		0%
1 star		0%

Share your thoughts with other customers

Write a customer review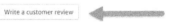

See all verified purchase reviews ›

Thank you from the bottom of our hearts for purchasing our pregnancy guide and we're hoping you enjoyed it right to the end! 🙏

SUPPORT THE KEEPING PARENTING REAL COMMUNITY

 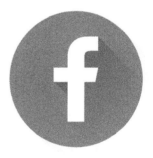

Join / share our Facebook Group here(access to all our free books)

Check out our **Customer Reviews & Testimonials!**

Keeping Parenting Real **Merchandise**and **Full Catalog**

Check out all our product reviews **here**

REFERENCES

Murkoff, Heidi & Mazel, Sharon. (2016). What to Expect When You're Expecting (Fifth Edition). Workman Publishing Company.

Mayo Clinic. (2018). Mayo Clinic Guide to a Healthy Pregnancy. (2nd Edition). Mayo Clinic Press.

Oster, Emily. (2014). Expecting Better: Why the Conventional Pregnancy Wisdom Is Wrong and What You Really Need to Know (First Edition). Penguin Books.

Simkin, Penny. (2018). Pregnancy, Childbirth, and the Newborn: The Complete Guide (Fifth Edition). Da Capo Lifelong Books.

Greenberg, Gary & Hayden, Jeannie. (2004). Be Prepared. Simon & Schuster.

Dais, Dawn. (2017). The Sh!t No One Tells You About Pregnancy: A Guide to Surviving Pregnancy, Childbirth, and Beyond (First Edition). Seal Press.

Schrock, Leslie. (2019). Bumpin': The Modern Guide to Pregnancy: Navigating the Wild, Weird, and Wonderful Journey From Conception Through Birth and Beyond (First Edition). Tiller Press

Brott, Armin & Ash, Jennifer. (2015). The Expectant Father: The Ultimate Guide for Dads-to-Be (Fourth Edition). Abbeville Press.

Kandis Lake, R. N. M. reviewed by L. A. (2021). Caffeine during pregnancy. BabyCenter. https://www.babycenter.com/pregnancy/diet-and-fitness/caffeine-during-pregnancy_3955.

Colleen, de B. (2020, December 11). How much water should you drink during pregnancy? What to Expect. https://www.whattoexpect.com/pregnancy/drink-enough-water/#tap.

Verywell, T. (n.d.). Try our recipe nutrition calculator. Verywell Fit. https://www.verywellfit.com/recipe-nutrition-analyzer-4157076.

Bonnie Rochman|Medically reviewed by Nancy Hudson, M. S. (n.d.). 8 things nutritionists wish you'd do during pregnancy. BabyCenter. https://www.babycenter.com/pregnancy/diet-and-fitness/pregnancy-food-diary_10395220.

Geddes, J. K. (2021, April 19). Food cravings and aversions during pregnancy. What to Expect. https://www.whattoexpect.com/pregnancy/symptoms-and-solutions/cravings-and-aversions.aspx.

Colleen de Bellefonds|Medically reviewed by Erin Hinga, M. S. (2021). Vegan and vegetarian pregnancy diets. BabyCenter. https://www.babycenter.com/pregnancy/diet-and-fitness/eating-a-vegetarian-diet-during-pregnancy_1313874.

RESOURCES

Mother.ly

Expectingscience.com

Womenshealth.gov/pregnancy

Babycenter.com

AmericanPregnancy.org

Thebump.com

Pregnancy.com

Healthline.com

Whattoexpect.com

Pregnancybirthbaby.org.au

Baby.com

Parents.com

Wikipedia.org/wiki/Pregnancy

Kidshealth.org

EatingWell.com

Image Credit: Shutterstock.com, Unsplash.com

Made in the USA
Las Vegas, NV
02 May 2022

48315410R00138